# Philosophical Studies Series

Volume 146

*Philosophical Studies Series* aims to provide a forum for the best current research in contemporary philosophy broadly conceived, its methodologies, and applications. Since Wilfrid Sellars and Keith Lehrer founded the series in 1974, the book series has welcomed a wide variety of different approaches, and every effort is made to maintain this pluralism, not for its own sake, but in order to represent the many fruitful and illuminating ways of addressing philosophical questions and investigating related applications and disciplines.

The book series is interested in classical topics of all branches of philosophy including, but not limited to:

- Ethics
- Epistemology
- Logic
- Philosophy of language
- Philosophy of logic
- Philosophy of mind
- Philosophy of religion
- Philosophy of science

Special attention is paid to studies that focus on:

- the interplay of empirical and philosophical viewpoints
- the implications and consequences of conceptual phenomena for research as well as for society
- philosophies of specific sciences, such as philosophy of biology, philosophy of chemistry, philosophy of computer science, philosophy of information, philosophy of neuroscience, philosophy of physics, or philosophy of technology; and
- contributions to the formal (logical, set-theoretical, mathematical, information-theoretical, decision-theoretical, etc.) methodology of sciences.

Likewise, the applications of conceptual and methodological investigations to applied sciences as well as social and technological phenomena are strongly encouraged.

*Philosophical Studies Series* welcomes historically informed research, but privileges philosophical theories and the discussion of contemporary issues rather than purely scholarly investigations into the history of ideas or authors. Besides monographs, *Philosophical Studies Series* publishes thematically unified anthologies, selected papers from relevant conferences, and edited volumes with a well-defined topical focus inside the aim and scope of the book series. The contributions in the volumes are expected to be focused and structurally organized in accordance with the central theme(s), and are tied together by an editorial introduction. Volumes are completed by extensive bibliographies.

The series discourages the submission of manuscripts that contain reprints of previous published material and/or manuscripts that are below 160 pages/88,000 words.

For inquiries and submission of proposals authors can contact the editor-in-chief Mariarosaria Taddeo via: mariarosaria.taddeo@oii.ox.ac.uk

More information about this series at https://link.springer.com/bookseries/6459

James F. Childress • Michael Quante
Editors

# Thick (Concepts of) Autonomy

## Personal Autonomy in Ethics and Bioethics

Springer

*Editors*
James F. Childress
University of Virginia
Charlottesville, VA, USA

Michael Quante
University of Münster
Münster, Germany

ISSN 0921-8599 ISSN 2542-8349 (electronic)
Philosophical Studies Series
ISBN 978-3-030-80990-4 ISBN 978-3-030-80991-1 (eBook)
https://doi.org/10.1007/978-3-030-80991-1



This Springer imprint is published by the registered company Springer Nature Switzerland AG
The registered company address is: Gewerbestrasse 11, 6330 Cham, Switzerland

# Preface

Many ethical theories and practices, particularly in domains such as biomedical ethics, incorporate minimal, formal, procedural conceptions of personal autonomy and autonomous decisions and actions. Over the last 30 years or so, concerns about the deficiencies and limitations of these "thin" conceptions have led to "thick" conceptions that highlight certain mental, corporeal, biographical, and social conditions of what it means to be a human person and that seek to enrich concepts of autonomy, with direct implications for ethical requirements to respect personal autonomy. The chapters in this book offer a wide range of perspectives, largely within an analytic philosophical approach, on both the elements of and the positive and negative relations between "thin" and "thick" concepts of autonomy as well as their relative roles and importance in ethics and bioethics.

It may be useful for readers to understand the logic of the overall structure of this volume even if, with that understanding, they autonomously chose to read the chapters in a different order. The first three chapters attend to key contested issues in conceptions of autonomy with particular reference to major philosophical contributors who have sought to frame and resolve these issues. Featured in all three of these chapters is the influential work of philosopher Harry Frankfurt who taught at Princeton University. Understanding and assessing Frankfurt's work is crucial for engaging in contemporary debates about conceptions of autonomy.

In the opening chapter, John Martin Fischer (University of California, Riverside) clarifies what autonomy is by examining what moral responsibility is *not*. Paying particular attention to Frankfurt's work, along with others, Fischer argues that failure to draw the appropriate distinction between "moral responsibility" and "autonomy" creates conceptual and normative difficulties. According to Fischer, "moral responsibility" refers to a minimal condition for rendering an agent an "apt target" for reactive attitudes, including moral blame. By contrast, "autonomy" indicates "a more robust notion of self-governance." It presupposes moral responsibility but is also more demanding. Although there is debate about how to specify what else is demanded, this roughly includes governance by the "real" or "true" self (or a designated set of goals or aims) in practical reasoning. An agent's failure to act in accordance with his or her true or real or designated self, perhaps because of weakness of will, can still be a free act in the sense required for moral responsibility, even though it falls short of autonomy. In short, the mental elements, particularly identification, that link choice and action are more robust for autonomy than for moral responsibility.

Joel Anderson (Utrecht University) rejects a common picture of Frankfurt's work on autonomy, contending that it does not seek to defend a moral theory of the person or of autonomy. Instead, what Frankfurt offers is a normatively thin ontology of autonomy, not a normative hierarchy of desires or wholeheartedness as a moral criterion. He distinguishes "persons" from "wantons," creatures who don't really care what they desire. According to Anderson, Frankfurt's central idea is that a necessary feature of the ontology of the will of persons is the capacity to be troubled by their desires. Anderson calls this the predicament of volitional reflexivity. In this interpretation, Frankfurt's goal is to provide an account of what would count as a successful response to this predicament, captured in the idea of volitional coherence and expressed in the language of "wholehearted" identification with some desires, that is, what one cares about. Refusals to face this predicament represent the passivity of non-persons ("wantons"). Volitional incoherence may threaten autonomy through ambivalence or disorientation. Anderson argues that Frankfurt's language of "wholeheartedness" and, more recently, "self-satisfaction" is too passive and excessively thin because it does not adequately incorporate self-understanding or making sense of the position one takes.

In Chap. 3 entitled "Determining Oneself and Determining One's Self," Thomas Schramme (University of Liverpool) exploits an ambiguity in the concept of self-determination. On the one hand, self-determination can mean to determine oneself in choices and actions; on the other hand, it can mean to determine one's self. In the second kind of self-determination, agents imagine alternative self-ideals to be actualized. Such a self-determination means not only to actualize a self but also to critically examine whether this self is the one that he or she wants to be or should be, where "should" is understood hypothetically, not categorically, because it is bound to the perspective of the person him- or herself. This normative conception of self-determination thus incorporates ideas of a right or good way to determine oneself. Developing his normative interpretation of self-determination by reference to three theorists (Harry Frankfurt, Thomas Hill Green, and John Stuart Mill), Schramme concludes by pulling together the "best elements" in their theories: "the proper way of self-determination consists in developing one's own human potentials as far as one oneself would like, in addition to realizing these potentials in decisions and actions."

Some internal and external conditions are important and even necessary for autonomy and its exercise in certain circumstances, as the next two chapters argue. Johann Ach (University of Münster) and Arnd Pollmann (Alice Salomon Hochschule Berlin) identify "the most fundamental personal condition for deciding or acting autonomously." They contend that, in contrast to elementary competence, this condition is too often neglected or, when recognized, rendered too demanding. In their formulation, the crucial self-relation in autonomous decisions and actions is the "triple-S-condition," consisting of "self confidence," "self-assertiveness," and "self-esteem." They argue that this triple-S-condition is necessary for autonomy and that any decision or action lacking it cannot appropriately be considered "autonomous." After describing the genesis and development of the triple-S-condition beginning in childhood and triple-S-susceptibility in later life, Ach and Pollmann draw some normative implications for ensuring and protecting the social relationships indispensable for acquiring and preserving the triple-S-condition.

In stressing that "autonomy is a cooperative enterprise in many ways," John Christman (Pennsylvania State University) focuses on the implications of respect for autonomy in relations in which mutual interactions help to establish or reestablish the autonomy of one or both of the agents and may constitute in part the exercise of their autonomy. An example of symmetrical power relations, featuring co-deliberation, involves romantic partners considering whether to have children, while an example of asymmetrical power relations is an aid worker helping a trauma victim regain autonomy. These "partnerships," in which interpersonal dynamics have a causal and constitutive relation to the establishment or exercise of autonomy, pose a challenge for the liberal sensibility of respect for autonomy. In such partnerships, the duty to respect another's autonomy should also take account of the ways that the interactions are constitutive as well as expressive of autonomy. Christman offers guidelines based on his socio-historical conception of autonomy. For instance, the obligation to respect the autonomy of others in relations that may influence the development of that autonomy must be diachronic in facilitating "the development of a practical identity which can be the basis of future judgments that would not be disturbed when considered in light of that very process of interaction and facilitation."

The next two chapters consider whether and to what extent mistaken beliefs or limited understanding can prevent decisions and actions from being autonomous. Viewing autonomy within "the family of metaphysical freedom terms" (including free action, free will, etc.), Alfred Mele (Florida State University) examines "actions distinctive of self-ruled or self-governed individuals" with attention to whether certain facts about beliefs might render an action non-autonomous. He uses several examples, including his well-known case of King George raising taxes 5% on the basis of the his advisors' provision of false information to him, to indicate the uncertainty about moving, along various dimensions, from apparently paradigmatic cases of different kinds of action, such as autonomous action, to other supposed instances of those kinds of action. Sometimes it is difficult to be confident about whether an action is autonomous or not (or intentional, or voluntary, or free or not). Nevertheless, Mele holds that an agent does not act autonomously if another agent has virtually complete control over the information going to the first agent and provides false information to the first agent who then acts on it. The first agent's action is heteronomous.

While there is widespread agreement that persons must understand what they are doing in order for their decisions or actions to be considered autonomous, there is little agreement or even much discussion in ethics or bioethics or other areas about *how much* understanding is required. In contrast to more robust, thicker accounts that require substantial understanding, James Stacey Taylor (The College of New

Jersey) concludes that "very little" understanding is actually required for autonomous decisions and actions. After first arguing that the moral value of autonomy does not undergird the ethical requirement to obtain a patient's informed consent in medical care, he then develops, against critics of this view, theoretical points about the sufficiency of a thin understanding for autonomous decisions and actions. In making his arguments, Taylor examines situations in which the acting agent's intentional description of the action is not how a neutral third party would describe it, and the agent's autonomous decisions and actions are of little value to him or her. He concludes that the minimalist account of understanding in autonomy is superior to more robust accounts.

The next two chapters consider negative and positive relations between certain "thick" conceptions of personal autonomy and respect for personal autonomy in decisions and actions. In Chap. 8 entitled "Is 'autonomy talk' misleading?" Thomas Gutmann (University of Münster) contends that the ongoing debate about autonomy would be greatly improved if the distinction between two concepts of autonomy were taken more seriously: (1) personal autonomy as a graded and at least moderately perfectionist ideal of the autonomous person, and (2) autonomy as right. He argues that these two concepts are independent and have different and even conflicting normative functions. Hence, it is important to treat them as separate, rather than to use quantitative characterizations such as "thinner" and "thicker" or "minimum" and "full" to distinguish them. To avoid confusion, Gutmann suggests that we call "autonomy as right" the "right to self-determination" or "authority," rather than "autonomy." This involves a threshold conception of competence, recognizes a binary, ontic status of persons who can make claims as moral equals, and focuses on the priority of right over the good (the latter including ideal concepts of autonomy). In questions about autonomy as authority in biomedical ethics or medical law, Gutmann insists, there is no place for "thick" concepts of autonomy, however important they may be in other contexts. No moral or legal consequences follow from not meeting thick concepts—a "bad" achiever of "thick" personal autonomy still has authority. According to Gutmann, any moral conception of autonomy is inadequate if it fails to account for the respect owed to autonomous agents whose equal moral right to hold views, make choices, and act in accord with their own values and rights should be acknowledged.

Focusing on respect for personal autonomy in bioethics—what Gutmann calls "autonomy as right" or as "authority"—James Childress (University of Virginia) explores several complexities of respecting autonomous choices by reference to the case of a 14-year-old boy who died after being allowed to refuse a necessary blood transfusion on religious grounds (the Jehovah's Witness tradition). Childress argues that some thicker concepts of autonomy, closely connected with relational autonomy, can direct our attention to aspects of respect for autonomy that are often neglected or underappreciated in bioethical theory and practice. In particular, they illuminate the interpretive complexity of respecting autonomous choices by attending to the relational context of individuals' decisions, respect for individuals' social-cultural beliefs and values, and the temporality of selves, as expressed in their past consent or future consent as well as in—and sometimes in contradiction to—their present consent or dissent. However, Childress' conclusion overlaps with Gutmann's: it is crucially important not to convert the illuminating and valuable insights from theories of relational autonomy into necessary conditions of autonomous choices and actions and hence of respect for autonomy.

The final two chapters consider whether, in certain contexts, different vulnerabilities to risk should affect judgments about whether an agent's decisions and actions are autonomous or non-autonomous. In autonomous authorization in bioethics, the notion of competence serves a "gate-keeping" function; it provides "an entrance ticket" that entitles patients to make authoritative treatment decisions in light of their non-medical values and preferences. Bettina Schöne-Seifert (University of Münster) considers whether the concept of mental competence, a key component in autonomous decision making and in informed consent to and refusal of medical procedures, varies according to the level of risk (i.e., the probability and magnitude of net harmful consequences) involved in the decision. A risk-related conception of competence, which assigns a "sliding scale" for competence based on the level of risk involved in the decision, is now widely used in practice and accepted by a number of bioethicists. However, Schöne-Seifert contends that this conception has two fatal flaws. On the one hand, paternalism can be buried in the concept of competence and can mask whether a patient's decision is overridden because of genuine incompetence or because of the risk of harm. On the other hand, a patient's self-authorization is devalued by attributing illusory autonomy to incompetent patients in low-risk situations. By contrast, Schöne-Seifert argues for a fixed concept of patients' decisional competence—the capacity to understand and appreciate—in the context of informed consent; this identifies a sufficiency threshold, independent of the level of risk involved in the decision.

In "Vulnerability, Exploitation, and Autonomy," Catriona Mackenzie (Macquarie University) challenges certain bioethical defenses of what intuitively appear to be exploitative commercial transactions, particularly organ sales and commercial surrogacy. These defenses combine a liberal analysis of exploitation with a libertarian analysis of autonomy. Mackenzie contends that the liberal analysis of exploitation sees these transactions as involving only two parties, thereby occluding the structural dimensions of exploitation. This occlusion then allows the transaction to be viewed in terms of libertarian autonomy. Mackenzie's approach instead pairs a vulnerability analysis of the transaction with a multidimensional, relational theory of autonomy, which together highlight the structural dimensions of exploitation and expose the myth-making that underlies claims that these forms of exploitation are actually autonomy-enhancing.

The volume concludes with "Outlook," some editorial reflections on its important contributions in illuminating, especially from the standpoint of analytic philosophy, the complexities and tensions in the distinctions and relations between "thick" and "thin" conceptions of autonomy and respect for autonomy. These reflections also note the volume's limits, which present challenging opportunities to develop broader perspectives on the autonomy of persons, decisions, and actions in at least three contexts. A first context is to broaden the range of philosophical traditions, beyond both analytic philosophy and western philosophy to encompass intercultural philosophy including dialogue with Asian and African traditions. A second context is the changing environment of autonomy, which includes challenges of an aging society, care for persons with dementia, information technologies, autonomous artificial systems (such as autonomous vehicles or weapons), and various kinds and means of personal enhancement. For many of these it is unclear and debatable whether proposed interventions strengthen, transform, or destroy personal autonomy. A third context includes tools from within and across particular sub-disciplines of philosophy, for example, not only ethics but also epistemology and philosophical anthropology, to name a few. This philosophical intra-disciplinarity and interdisciplinarity also needs to be accompanied by rigorous research findings related to autonomy from relevant social, biological, and other sciences.

Most of the chapters in this volume were initially prepared for an international conference on "Thick (Concepts of) Autonomy?" organized by the Centre for Advanced Study in Bioethics at Westfälische Wilhelms-Universität in Münster, Germany, in October 2012. These original papers were then thoroughly revised based on the discussions at and after the conference, and supplemented by additional contributions. This rich examination of autonomy within the broad analytic philosophical tradition is an international undertaking, with contributors from Germany, the United States, the Netherlands, the United Kingdom, and Australia.

As editors, we thank the authors of these chapters for their important contributions to on-going debates about how best to characterize personal autonomy and autonomous decisions and actions, the elements and the advantages and disadvantages of "thin" and "thick" versions of these concepts, the various positive and negative relations between these versions, and their implications for respect for autonomy in both ethics and bioethics.

Charlottesville, VA, USA James F. Childress

Münster, Germany Michael Quante
May 2021

# Contents

# Chapter 1
# What Moral Responsibility is Not

**John Martin Fischer**

**Abstract** Moral responsibility and autonomy are closely related structurally and contentwise: they are both members of the "freedom family". Here I argue that because of these similarities, they are often conflated or at least not carefully separated, and that this has resulted in confusions in important contemporary debates. Autonomy and moral responsibility involve the agent's identification with the sources of her actions; but autonomy-identification is more robust than responsibility-identification.

## 1.1 Introduction

Over the years I have noted that there appear to be two separate–but often conflated–notions: moral responsibility and autonomy. In previous work, I have sought to distinguish these notions and to sketch some difficulties that can arise if they are not distinguished appropriately.[1] Here I shall further explore aspects of the distinction between moral responsibility and autonomy. I shall argue that Harry Frankfurt's focus has shifted subtly from moral responsibility to autonomy over the course of his career, and I wish to identify some additional examples–from the work of such influential philosophers as Gary Watson, Charles Taylor, David Velleman, and Michael Bratman in which the failure (in at least some authors) to keep these closely related notions distinct has vitiated the analysis of the phenomena.[2]

[1] See John Martin Fischer (2010, 2012).

[2] I do not mean to claim that all of these philosophers themselves have been insufficiently attentive to the distinction; some of them have been explicit in making the distinction. My main point is that

J. M. Fischer (✉)
University of California, Riverside, CA, USA
e-mail: John.fischer@ucr.edu



J. F. Childress, M. Quante (eds.), *Thick (Concepts of) Autonomy*, Philosophical Studies Series 146, https://doi.org/10.1007/978-3-030-80991-1_1

## 1.2 Frankfurt

In his early articles, Harry Frankfurt's fundamental focus was on distinguishing two kinds of freedom—"freedom to do otherwise" and "acting freely"—and arguing that acting freely (properly understood) is both compatible with causal determinism and all the freedom required for moral responsibility. He thus construed his contributions in these early papers as squarely within the realm of the traditional debates in metaphysics about the relationships between causal determinism, freedom, and moral responsibility.

In his 1969 essay, "Alternate Possibilities and Moral Responsibility," Frankfurt is clearly addressing those who have thought that freedom to do otherwise is required for moral responsibility. He argues that such freedom is not required for moral responsibility, and thus we might be able to make progress on the traditional metaphysical debates, which tended to focus on the relationship between causal determinism and freedom to do otherwise. If Frankfurt is correct here, we can side-step these debates and attend to whether "acting freely" is compatible with causal determinism.[3]

Now Frankfurt goes on in his 1971 paper, "Freedom of the Will and the Concept of a Person," to give an account of "acting freely" and to explore aspects of its relationship to causal determinism. He first argues that his theory of freedom of the will can meet two conditions that various other accounts cannot: it can account for our disinclination to attribute such freedom to members of other species and it can show why freedom of the will is desirable. Frankfurt goes on to say:

> It is generally supposed that, in addition to satisfying the two conditions I have mentioned, a satisfactory theory of the freedom of the will necessarily provides an analysis of one of the conditions of moral responsibility. The most common recent approach to the problem of understanding the freedom of the will has been, indeed, to inquire what is entailed by the assumption that someone is morally responsible for what he has done. In my view, however, the relation between moral responsibility and the freedom of the will has been very widely misunderstood. It is not true that a person is morally responsible for what he has done only if his will was free when he did it.
>
> … For the assumption that a person is morally responsible for what he has done does not entail that the person was in a position to have whatever will he wanted. This assumption *does* entail that the person did what he did freely… It is a mistake, however, to believe that someone acts freely only when he is free to do whatever he wants…(1971, pp. 18–19)

Frankfurt reiterates in the concluding section of the paper the point that the sort of freedom that involves access to alternative possibilities (freedom to will or do otherwise) is *not* required for moral responsibility. Rather, according to Frankfurt, the freedom-relevant requirement for moral responsibility is acting freely, and–in the view presented in "Freedom of the Will and the Concept of a Person"–it suffices for

---

a proper evaluation of some of their work will require care in distinguishing moral responsibility from autonomy.

[3] For further discussion and a defense of Frankfurt's strategy here, see: John Martin Fischer (2002), reprinted in John Martin Fischer (2006, pp. 124–142).

acting freely that one identifies with the particular first-order desire that moves one to action via the formation of a second-order volition (i.e., a second-order preference to act in accordance with a certain first-order desire). Here it is in virtue of the second-order volition that one "identifies" with the relevant first-order desire, in the sense of "identification" involved in moral responsibility. We can say that Frankfurt is here answering the question of what must be added to merely acting on desire to get to the kind of freedom linked to (and, more specifically, entailed by) moral responsibility; the answer is that one must in a distinctive way "identify" with the desire, and this identification consists in forming an appropriate second-order volition.

Frankfurt concludes the paper with ruminations on the relationship between his account of freedom of the will and the traditional metaphysical worries about the relationship between such freedom and causal determinism:

> My conception of the freedom of the will appears to be neutral with regard to the problem of determinism. It seems conceivable that it should be causally determined that a person is free to want what he wants to want. If this is conceivable, then it might be causally determined that a person enjoys a free will…(1971, p. 20)

Whatever else Frankfurt had in mind in putting forward his "hierarchical" account of acting freely, he certainly sought in his early papers to make contributions to the traditional metaphysical debates about determinism, free will, and moral responsibility.[4]

But I would contend that, beginning with Frankfurt's "Identification and Externality," there is a subtle shift in Frankfurt's aim—a shift that Frankfurt himself does not explicitly note.[5] Perhaps, although this is difficult to ascertain, Frankfurt did not even realize that he was shifting his target of analysis from the notion of freedom that is a condition for moral responsibility to a rather different notion of freedom. But whether or not Frankfurt recognized this shift, I wish to argue that he did indeed change his focus of attention. And others followed suit.

As noted above, in "Freedom of the Will and the Concept of a Person," Frankfurt employs the term, "identification", to refer to a psychic element that must be added to action on a first-order desire to get to "acting freely", the freedom-relevant condition for moral responsibility. Further, this condition is arguably consistent with causal determinism; at least it is not in tension with causal determinism in the way that freedom to do otherwise is. But in "Identification and Externality," I do not find any uses of the terms "causal determinism" and "moral responsibility"; nor do I find any instances of "freedom". The focus here is not on the traditional metaphysical problems concerning causal determinism, freedom, and moral responsibility; the

[4] In his 2002 article "Reply to John Martin Fischer," Frankfurt further elaborated and explained his views on the traditional problem of the relationship between causal determinism and moral responsibility. Here he explained that his goal has been to address certain objections to compatibilism, although he remains officially neutral about the compatibility of causal determinism and moral responsibility insofar as he is not sufficiently confident that causal determination is consistent with being active (rather than passive): p. 29.

[5] Frankfurt (1976); reprinted in Frankfurt (1988, pp. 58–68).

focus is on something else—something perhaps closely related to the traditional issues, for which Frankfurt also employs the term, "identification".

Roughly speaking, Frankfurt says that corresponding to the distinction between action and mere movement of the body, there is a distinction between being identified with a "passion" (or mental element) and being alienated from a passion (or mental element); that is, there is a distinction between a mental feature's being "internal" to one's mind or in a certain special sense "one's own" and its being "external" to oneself in this special sense, although also in a different sense one's own. As Frankfurt puts it:

> The problem of attribution or of externality with regard to bodily movements is to explain what differentiates a movement that a person makes from a mere happening in the history of his body. The corresponding problem with regard to psychic phenomena concerns the nature of identification: what does it mean for a person to be identified with one rather than with another of two passions (or whatever), both of which are in the gross literal sense his? Each of these problems is, in its own realm, both fundamental and frustratingly recalcitrant. (1976, p. 251)

In this paper Frankfurt makes a distinction that is important to the subsequent development of his views—a distinction between two desires that fit into the same ordering, as it were, and two desires that do not fit into the same ordering. When two desires—say, a desire to see a concert and a desire to see a film—fit into the same ordering, the agent's challenge is simply to figure out which desire should have priority within the single ordering. On the other hand, one might have a conscious desire to compliment a friend on a recent accomplishment but also a (perhaps) unconscious desire to insult him out of jealousy. As Frankfurt puts it:

> When a person suffers a conflict of [this] kind, his problem is not to assign one desire that he feels to a lower position than another on a single scale. It is to reject one of the desires that he feels altogether. Conflicts between conscious and unconscious desires are typically of this kind, but both of the conflicting desires may well remain conscious. … The conflict is not one to be resolved by *ordering* the conflicting desires, in other words, but by *rejecting* one of them. In rejecting the desire to injure his acquaintance, presuming that this is what he does, the person withdraws himself from it. He places the rejected desire outside the scope of his preferences, so that it is not a candidate for satisfaction at all. Although he may continue to experience the rejected desire as occurring in his mental history, the person brings it about in this way that its occurrence is an external one. The desire is then no longer to be attributed strictly to him, even though it may well persist or recur as an element of his experience. (1976, p. 250)

Here, then, Frankfurt's target of analysis seems to be something a bit different from the notion of freedom linked to moral responsibility. Here "identification" is supposed to pick out a process whereby certain of one's goals or aims are thought to be more closely associated with oneself—these goals are "internal" to oneself in a special way—a way in which other goals, although one's own, are not. In using "identification" to pick out the process whereby some goals or aims become more truly one's own, Frankfurt is subtly shifting his target of analysis.

In the early papers, "identification" was employed to denote the mental element that is to be added to mere action on the basis of a particular first-order desire to get to "acting freely" (the sort of freedom implicated in moral responsibility). Again, I do not know if Frankfurt himself was at the time of writing "Identification and Externality" aware of the shift, and the fact that the target of analysis has subtly changed can easily be missed by a reader, especially given that the same term, "identification", is employed by Frankfurt in the 1971 paper and also "Identification and Externality", published in 1976.

In his subsequent work, Frankfurt seems to be increasingly interested in the notion of identification that plays a role in specifying a set of aims or goals more closely associated with the self, rather than the more minimal notion of identification that is (putatively) part of the freedom-relevant condition for moral responsibility. I introduce a bit of technical terminology here to simplify the exposition.[6] That is, I shall use the term, "moral responsibility", to refer to a more minimal condition, in which an agent is (for example) an apt target for the reactive attitudes (on the Strawsonian way of interpreting the nature of moral responsibility). And I shall use the term "autonomy" to refer to a more robust notion of self-governance, which presupposes moral responsibility but requires more. What more is required is contentious and difficult to specify, but roughly it involves governance by the "real" or "true" self as regards practical reasoning, that is, governance by a special or designated "part" of the self or (slightly less metaphorically) set of aims and goals. Although Frankfurt does not make this distinction explicitly, or employ the terms, "moral responsibility" and "autonomy" as above, I contend that the distinction is important. Further, I claim that in his later work Frankfurt's main (although not exclusive) focus is on autonomy, rather than mere moral responsibility.

In his later work, beginning perhaps with his essay, "The Importance of What We Care About," Frankfurt is primarily interested in giving an account of "caring" and explicating the role of caring in understanding our agency and in explaining normativity (the way in which considerations become *reasons for action* for agents, on one way of conceptualizing these matters).[7] On the view of caring defended by Frankfurt, identification—understood as the formation of a second-order preference to act in accordance with a certain first-order desire–plays a role, but there are additional requirements (that is, requirements in addition to those for acting freely). These requirements involve the idea that one cares about things and persons only if one has a relatively stable and long-term commitment to the targets of the attitude of caring. So, for example, if one finds the first-order desire in question "flagging" or becoming less strong, one is disposed to take measures to refresh it. As Frankfurt puts is:

> A person who cares about something is, as it were, invested in it. He *identifies* himself with what he cares about in the sense that he makes himself vulnerable to losses and susceptible to benefits depending upon whether what he cares about is diminished or enhanced. (1988, p. 83)

On Frankfurt's view, when one cares about something, one has a higher-order attitude that the relevant first-order desire "not be extinguished or abandoned"

---

[6] Here I follow Fischer (2012).

[7] Frankfurt (1982); reprinted in Frankfurt (1988, pp. 80–94). Subsequent references will be to the reprinted version.

(Frankfurt 1999a, p. 161). About someone who cares about attending a concert, Frankfurt says:

> … his caring about going to the concert implies that he is disposed to support and sustain his desire to go to it even after he has decided that he prefers to satisfy another desire instead. Forgoing the concert would frustrate his first-order desire to attend the concert. In itself, on the other hand, it would fail to touch the higher-order desire—which he might or might not have—that this first-order desire not be extinguished or abandoned. His caring about the concert would essentially consist in his having and identifying with a higher-order desire of this kind.
>
> … Whether the person cares about the concert is not fundamentally, then, a question either of how enthusiastic he *feels* about going to it or of how beneficial he *believes* or *expects* going to it would be. No doubt beliefs, feelings, and expectations of those kinds *do*, in many situations, more or less reliably indicate whether a person considers something to be important to him. What is at the heart of the matter, however, is not a condition of *feeling* or of *belief* or of *expectation* but of *will*. The question of whether a person cares about something pertains essentially to whether he is *committed* to his desire for it in the way that I have suggested, or whether he is willing and prepared to give the desire up and to have it excluded from the order of preferences. (1999a, p. 161)

What, then, is the importance of what we care about? In my view, Frankfurt takes it that what we care about specifies the "true" or "real" or "designated" self, as regards practical reasoning: the set of aims and goals that specify what is more closely associated with the agent and thus would help to define autonomy (self-governance). As Frankfurt puts it, one *identifies* oneself with what one cares about; caring is an element that helps to specify what one identifies oneself with in the sense of a set of aims or goals that are more truly one's own.

Frankfurt goes on to develop an account of love that builds on his account of caring; on this view, love involves caring about someone's interests for their own sake and also not being able to avoid or resist so caring. Thus, for Frankfurt, love is a species of caring that is characterized by "volitional necessity" (Frankfurt 1999b). Another role played by caring in Frankfurt's overall framework is that it generates normativity; we have reasons for action—including reasons for being moral—only to the extent that we *care* about the relevant action and, indeed, about morality. The "true self" is the self that explains our reasons for action, and for Frankfurt that it is a matter of what you care about.[8]

To take stock, I claim that Frankfurt was not always careful to distinguish between moral responsibility, which was the primary focus of his early work (in particular, the famous 1969 and 1971 papers in *The Journal of Philosophy*) and autonomy, which was the primary (although not exclusive) focus of his later work. The crucial notion of identification plays a role in Frankfurt's accounts of both moral responsibility and autonomy, and this common element (and term) might have (at least in some places) made it more difficult—for Frankfurt and other theorists—to separate the phenomena. But it is analytically important to distinguish the notions of moral responsibility and autonomy.[9] For example, it seems clear that one

[8] See, for example, Frankfurt (2004) and Frankfurt (2006).

[9] For additional argumentation for this point, see Fischer (2012).

could act in a "weak-willed" manner, that is, against the dictates of one's "true" or "real" or "designated" self. In such a case, one would (or could) be morally responsible and yet one would not be acting autonomously. Moral responsibility is the "gateway" to autonomy, but it is less demanding; one can be morally responsible but not self-governing in the way required by autonomy.

I am not sure whether Frankfurt was aware of the shift in his focus. Here it might be helpful to consider the beginning of the entry on "Mission Creep" in Wikipedia:

> Mission creep is the expansion of a project or mission beyond its original goals, often after initial successes. The term often implies a certain disapproval of newly adopted goals by the user of the term. Mission creep is usually considered undesirable due to the dangerous path of each success breeding more ambitious attempts, only stopping when a final, often catastrophic, failure occurs. The term was originally applied exclusively to military operations, but has recently been applied to many different fields. The phrase first appeared in articles concerning the UN Peacekeeping mission during the Somali Civil War in the Washington Post on April 15, 1993 and in the New York Times on October 10, 1993. (Wikipedia 2011)

A salient example of mission creep relates to the United States policy surrounding the war in Iraq (launched by George W. Bush). Originally, the mission was to find and destroy the "weapons of mass destruction" that were allegedly possessed by Iraq (under the leadership of Saddam Hussein). When such weapons were not found, the United States explicitly changed the mission to one involving the elimination of a tyrant and the building of a reasonably stable "democracy" in the region of the Middle East.

Mission creep can then come in (at least) two varieties. In one form, the mission is explicitly (or fairly explicitly) reevaluated and changed openly. In another form, the mission does in fact change, but the change is not explicitly recognized and/or acknowledged. This kind of mission creep might be called "mission drift", and I would suggest that mission drift arguably, at least, characterizes Frankfurt's work on agency (and related topics) over the years.

I must concede that there are elements even in Frankfurt's early work on these topics that suggest that he might have in mind as the target of his analysis something closer to autonomy than moral responsibility. Also, even in his later work—work that focuses primarily on developing accounts of caring, love, and normativity—Frankfurt does indeed come back to the role of identification in the traditional metaphysical disputes. He says:

> But suppose that we are doing what we want to do, that our motivating first-order desire to perform the action is exactly the desire by which we want our action to be motivated, and that there is no conflict in us between this motive and any desire at any higher order. In other words, suppose we are thoroughly wholehearted both in what we are doing and in what we want. Then there is no respect in which we are being violated or defeated or coerced. Neither our desires nor the conduct to which they lead are imposed upon us without our consent or against our will. We are acting just as we want, and our motives are just what we want them to be. Then so far as I can see, we have on that occasion all the freedom for which finite creatures can reasonably hope. Indeed, I believe that we have as much freedom as it is possible for us even to conceive.
>
> Notice that this has nothing to do with whether our actions, our desires, or our choices are causally determined. The widespread conviction among thoughtful people that there is

> a radical opposition between free will and determinism is, on this account, a red herring. (2006, pp. 15–16)

Whereas I contend that the thrust of Frankfurt's efforts in his early work seeks to analyze moral responsibility (rather than autonomy) and that a subtle shift—a "mission drift"—occurs over the course of Frankfurt's career, Benjamin Mitchell-Yellin (2012) has suggested that Frankfurt's work has always had elements that address each of these related notions. That is, Mitchell-Yellin claims that there has not so much been a change in focus over the course of Frankfurt's career, but that Frankfurt has always been concerned with both notions, although he has not always been sufficiently careful about distinguishing them. For my purposes here it does not really matter whether the Mission Drift thesis or some alternative, such as a Mish-mash Thesis, is true; what is most important is the contention that there are two closely related but importantly different notions—moral responsibility and autonomy—that are not always distinguished with sufficient care in Frankfurt's work.

I should point out that Frankfurt has indeed shown an awareness of the distinction in question (which I have marked by "moral responsibility" and "autonomy"). In the Preface to his 1988 collection, *The Importance of What We Care About*, Frankfurt says:

> So far as freedom is concerned, it is of course true that freedom is commonly understood to be a necessary condition of moral responsibility. Moreover, the nature of freedom is often investigated, as in several efforts of my own, in the light of that particular connection. On the other hand, I do not think that it is mainly for the sake of moral responsibility that we care as much as we do about being free. Nor am I convinced that it is possible to illuminate what it means for us to be free only if we begin by construing freedom specifically as a condition that being morally responsible requires. (1988, p. viii)

I agree with Frankfurt that it is not *only* in light of our interest in moral responsibility that we are concerned about freedom, and it might even be correct that it is not "mainly" for the sake of moral responsibility that we are interested in freedom. And I certainly agree with Frankfurt here that there are various routes to illumination about freedom; it is not true that the only such route is via reflection on the conditions for moral responsibility. No worries thus far. But I would still insist that it is analytically important to distinguish moral responsibility from autonomy; freedom as it relates to moral responsibility need not be the same as freedom as it relates to autonomy, and failing to keep the notions of freedom separate can lead to confusions and difficulties.

As above, note that one can fail to act in accordance with one's "true", "real", or "designated" self and yet act freely in the sense relevant to moral responsibility. That is, one can presumably freely fail to pursue any of the set of aims and goals specified by one's account of autonomy as more closely associated with oneself; some such cases might well be cases in which one is morally responsible for one's behavior. Thus, it is important to distinguish moral responsibility from autonomy. An account of autonomy that is problematic—that in some way fails to capture the "true" or "real" self as regards practical reasoning—would not *thereby* be problematic as an account of moral responsibility. This is my point, and it is completely compatible with the contentions that we do not care about freedom solely or even mainly because of its relationship to moral responsibility and that it is not true that the only route to illumination of freedom is through reflection on the conditions for moral responsibility.

## 1.3 Other Theorists: Taylor, Watson, and Velleman

### *1.3.1 Taylor*

In his famous paper, "Responsibility for Self," it emerges that Charles Taylor interprets Frankfurt as primarily seeking to give an account of what I have called, "autonomy", rather than moral responsibility (even though Taylor employs the term "responsibility" for the target phenomenon). He begins the paper as follows:

> What is the notion of responsibility which is bound up with our conception of a person or self? Is there a sense in which the human agent is responsible for himself which is part of our very conception of the self?
>
> This is certainly a commonly held idea, among 'ordinary men' as well as among philosophers. … Frankfurt has made the point (*J. Phil.*, Jan. 1971) that a person is more than just a subject of desires, of choices, even of deliberation; that we attribute to persons the ability to form 'second-order desires'; to want to be moved by certain desires, or 'second-order volitions': to want certain first order desires to be the ones which move them to action.
>
> If we think of what we are as defined by our goals, by what we desire to encompass or maintain, then a person on this view is one who can raise the question: Do I really want to be what I now am? (i.e., have the desires and goals I now have). In other words, beyond the *de facto* characterization of the subject by his goals, desires, and purposes, a person is a subject who can pose the *de jure* question: is this the kind of being I ought to be, or really want to be? There is as Frankfurt puts it a 'capacity for reflective self-evaluation'… manifest in the formation of second-order desires (*J. Phil.*, 7). (1976, p. 281)

Taylor contends that Frankfurt's apparatus, as it stands, is too weak to capture the pertinent kind of reflective self-evaluation, of which he seeks to give his own account. Taylor's account of the putatively required reflective self-evaluation involves what he calls "strong evaluation", rather than "simple weighing" of alternatives. For Taylor, a strong evaluator can offer articulate explanations of the superiority of one course of action over another, where these courses of action are experienced as incommensurable. It is perhaps not too much of a distortion to say that, on Taylor's view, the required kind of reflective self-evaluation involves the capacity to employ and articulate something like deontological, and not mere consequentialist, evaluations of courses of action.

I claim that Taylor interprets Frankfurt's 1971 account as seeking to specify what I above called "autonomy", rather than moral responsibility. That is, Taylor invites us to "think of what we are as defined by our goals", and then gives what he takes to be a more refined and plausible account of how to pick out these goals—the goals more closely associated with the person in question. Here Taylor is interpreting the capacity to step back from one's first-order desires and to identify with one of them via the formation of a second-order volition as part of a project of specifying the "designated" set of aims or goals—the "true" or "real" self, as it plays a role in autonomy.[10]

As above, it is perhaps unclear just how Frankfurt was interpreting his account, even in his 1971 paper. But it is at least worth noting that one of Frankfurt's avowed aims in that paper was to address the traditional metaphysical issues pertaining to the relationship between casual determinism, freedom, and moral responsibility. It is then not so surprising that Frankfurt gave a rather "minimalist" account of identification in the 1971 paper, and emphasized that the relevant second-order volition need not be based on any specific, substantive sort of reflection, including rational reflection of any sort.

Frankfurt's claim here would be more appropriate if one's fundamental aim were to give an account of moral responsibility, rather than autonomy. Further, it seems to me that Taylor's suggestion is more appropriate as an account of autonomy than of moral responsibility. For certainly one could be morally responsible for a choice that does not in any way spring from strong evaluation; here one might well be failing to act autonomously and failing to act in accordance with some norm pertaining to our agency and even personhood, broadly conceived; but one would not thereby fail to be morally responsible. Or so I would suggest, and it seems best to leave this open as a theoretical possibility.

Perhaps Taylor would wish to maintain that the capacity for strong evaluation is a requirement for moral responsibility, even when strong evaluation is not exhibited in a particular case (or in the causal sequence leading to a particular choice and bit of behavior). This may be true, but it is rather delicate and difficult to evaluate such a claim. I do not here wish to dispute this sort of position. That is, it may well be that an agent is morally responsible only if he has at least the capacity to engage in a certain sort of rational self-reflection.[11] But I would simply point out that acting freely, in the sense relevant to being morally responsible for a particular choice and bit of behavior, does not require that one exhibit or display such reflection either at the time of the behavior in question or along the causal sequence to it.

---

[10] In his work on Frankfurt, it is obvious that Jan Bransen (1996, 2000) interprets Frankfurt in a similar fashion. Bransen emphasizes the distinction between "identifying with" and "identifying as", and he contends that the proper interpretation of Frankfurt employs "identifying as". According to this approach, when an agent identifies as such and such, he picks out such and such as an "alternative of oneself". So, on this picture, identification is not about selecting a certain designated mental element, but, rather, about defining oneself in a certain way.

[11] For a very thoughtful exploration of this (and related issues), see: Andrew Eshleman (2004).

### 1.3.2 Watson

Gary Watson has offered an insightful and influential critique of Frankfurt, and also an alternative account of free action, in his paper, "Free Agency".[12] Watson criticizes Frankfurt's hierarchical model, and he endorses a non-hierarchical model in which there are different "sources" of behavior—motives and values. Put simply, on Watson's approach, one acts freely to the extent that one harmonizes these different sources; that is, an individual acts freely insofar as he is motivated by his values. On this view, unfreedom stems from a discordance between values and motivation.

Watson says:

> … It is not easy to give a nontrivial account of the sense of 'to value' in question. … We might say that an agent's values consist in those principles and ends which he—in a cool and non-self-deceptive moment—articulates as definitive of the good, fulfilling, and defensible life. That most people have articulate 'conceptions of the good,' coherent life-plans, *systems* of ends, and so on, is of course something of a fiction. Yet we all have more or less long-term aims and normative principles that we are willing to defend. It is such things as these that are to be identified as our values. (p. 91)

Unfortunately, Watson does not say much more about the crucial notions, "good" and "defensible"; for example, from what perspective and to whom is the conception of the good and fulfilling life to be defended? In any case, Watson continues:

> The *valuational system* of an agent is that set of considerations which, when combined with his factual beliefs (and probability estimates), yields judgments of the form: the thing for me to do in these circumstances, all things considered, is *a*. To ascribe free agency to a being presupposes it to be a being that makes judgments of this sort. To be this sort of being, one must assign values to alternative states of affairs, that is, rank them in terms of worth.
>
> The *motivational system* of an agent is that set of considerations which move him to action. We identify his motivational system by identifying what motivates him. The possibility of unfree action consists in the fact that an agent's valuational system and motivational system may not completely coincide. Those systems harmonize to the extent that what determines the agent's all-things-considered judgments also determines his actions. (p. 91)

Watson at least *appears* to claim here that one acts freely if and only if one's values and motivations are in alignment. (He does not here discuss the possibility that one's values do not specify a unique action or that perhaps one's valuational system contains elements that are incommensurable.) Perhaps a more accurate way of formulating Watson's claim is: one acts freely if and only if one is moved to act by a desire because of the worth of its object.[13]

As with Taylor, Watson criticizes Frankfurt's account of freedom as being too "minimalist" or austere. Watson holds that merely invoking desires, even desires of higher orders, does not give one enough resources adequately to analyze the relevant kind of freedom. According to Watson, one must add values to the

---

[12] Watson (1975); reprinted in *Moral Responsibility* (1986), ed. Fischer, pp. 81–96. All references will be to the reprinted version.

[13] I am indebted to Benjamin Mitchell-Yellin for this suggestion.

psychological mix. But now note that Watson faces an obvious problem of accommodating weak-willed agency (here understood as free action against one's values). Insofar as Watson appears to define free action as simply a harmony between value and motivation, and unfree action as a lack of such a harmony, he would appear to leave no room for genuinely free but weak action. And this is a deep problem for Watson's view.[14]

The problem here stems from requiring too close a connection between value and motivation. Of course, as in the analysis of Taylor above, we could interpret Watson as seeking to give an account of autonomy, rather than moral responsibility. Alternatively, again as in the discussion of Taylor, we could loosen the connection posited by Watson to simply require, for free action, that the agent have the ability or power to achieve a harmony between value and motive, even if he does not actually achieve this harmony. This would be parallel to the interpretation of Taylor as requiring, for moral responsibility, merely the capacity to engage in strong evaluation, rather than the actual exercise of such evaluation in the sequence leading to the behavior under consideration.

In evaluating Watson's approach, as in the case of Taylor's model, it is crucial to distinguish between moral responsibility (and its associated freedom) and autonomy (and its associated freedom). One can exercise a robust kind of freedom, in virtue of which one is fully morally responsible, even when one does not act in accordance with one's strong evaluations or one's values. We have to leave conceptual space for this possibility. If we do not distinguish moral responsibility from autonomy, we are in jeopardy of collapsing the space of possibilities, and in so doing, conflating issues and vitiating our analyses of related—but distinct—agency phenomena.

### *1.3.3 Velleman and Bratman*

In "What Happens When Someone Acts?", David Velleman offers an interesting critique of Frankfurt.[15] He says:

> Suppose that I have a long-anticipated meeting with an old friend for the purpose of resolving some minor difference; but that as we talk, his offhand comments provoke me to raise my voice in progressively sharper replies, until we part in anger. Later reflection leads me to realize that accumulated grievances had crystallized in my mind, during the weeks before our meeting, into a resolution to sever our friendship over the matter at hand, and that this resolution is what gave the hurtful edge to my remarks. In short, I may conclude that desires of mine caused a decision, which in turn caused the corresponding behaviour; and I may acknowledge that these mental states were thereby exerting their normal motivational force,

[14] In contrast to Frankfurt, Watson has admitted that weakness of the will constitutes a challenge for his view, and he has grappled with this problem in numerous subsequent papers, including: Watson (1977, 1987, 1999, and 2003).

[15] Velleman (1992); reprinted in *Perspectives on Moral Responsibility* (1993), eds. John Martin Fischer and Mark Ravizza, pp. 188–210. Subsequent citations will be to the reprinted version.

> unabetted by any strange perturbation or compulsion. But do I necessarily think that I made the decision or that I executed it? Surely, I can believe that the decision, though genuinely motivated by my desires, was thereby induced in me but not formed by me; and I can believe that it was genuinely executed in my behaviour but executed, again, without my help. Indeed, viewing the decision as directly motivated by my desires, and my behavior as directly governed by the decision, is precisely what leads to the thought that as my words became more shrill, it was my resentment speaking, not I. (pp. 191–192)

Velleman is here criticizing the notion that one can give a proper analysis of action that reflects the true self—where the agent really stands—simply by employing the resources of desire, belief, and "standard causation", even supplemented by Frankfurt's notion of "decisive commitment" (Frankfurt 1987). It should be evident that Velleman is interested in something different from mere moral responsibility, or so at least I would suggest.[16] Indeed, it seems to me that the individual depicted in Velleman's story can legitimately be held morally responsible for his "decision" to sever his relationship with his friend, just as one can be held morally responsible for various habitual, unreflective, and or even subconsciously-motivated behavior. One is morally responsible for severing one's relationship with one's friend, even if it does not stem from one's "true self".

Insofar as we share Velleman's intuition about such a case that the individual is not fully and robustly involved, we might say that, although the individual is fully morally responsible for severing his relationship with his friend, he does not do so autonomously. His behavior in severing the relationship thus does not reflect a more robust participation or involvement of the self. It is not evident to me, from the story as told by Velleman, that this is indeed so. Perhaps Velleman's view about the case stems from an excessively intellectualist theory of the relevant aspects of the self.[17] But we can imagine that the story is filled in so that it is more congenial to Velleman's conclusion. Even so, such a case would at best show that a Frankfurtian model would not provide a fully adequate account of autonomy; it would not follow that such a model could not provide an adequate account of the more minimal notion of moral responsibility. Failing to distinguish these two potential targets of analysis could then lead to analytical difficulties. If one concluded from a story such as Velleman's that Frankfurt has given an inadequate account of moral responsibility, this would be a mistake.

Similarly, consider Michael Bratman's example:

> Perhaps I think it strictly better to be a person who forgives and turns the other check [*sic*] but nevertheless, in a kind of self-indulgence, allow into my life a willingness to express reactive anger. Though this role of my desire to express my anger diverges from my relevant evaluative judgments, it is not a desire I reject or disown. ... So, value judgment is one thing, and ownership another. (2003, reprinted in 2007; quotation on p. 144 of 2007)

Bratman is here offering a critique of Watson's "Platonic" model of the "true" self, according to which one is identified (as this notion figures in an analysis of

---

[16] Velleman agrees: see note 11, p. 192 of paper as reprinted in Fischer and Ravizza, eds., *Perspectives on Moral Responsibility*.

[17] I am indebted to Justin Coates for this point.

autonomy) with those desires endorsed by one's evaluative commitments. My contention is that, whatever is correct about the true self and autonomy, we can consider Bratman morally responsible for acting from anger (in the case as Bratman describes it). So if one concluded from a story such as Bratman's that Watson has given an inadequate account of moral responsibility, this would be a mistake.

## 1.4 Conclusion: What Moral Responsibility is Not

In the last 40 years or so there has been a tremendous explosion of literature in what has come to be called "agency theory". Some of this work has focused on freedom—freedom to do otherwise, free action, and acting freely. Freedom is thought (by many, although not all) to be a condition on moral responsibility, although the specific notion of freedom in question is a matter of controversy. But freedom—of some kind or another—is also a key feature of something related to, but different from, moral responsibility; I have called this more robust thing, "autonomy", because it involves a kind of self-governance, where the "self" is perhaps a more robust notion than the corresponding element in moral responsibility.

Various philosophers who have written on these subjects have used different terms for their target of analysis. Some have indeed employed "moral responsibility" to pick out the target of their inquiry, and others have used "autonomy". Still others have used terms such as "agency *par excellence*" and "agency at its best". Some have talked of behavior that is guided by mental elements that have "agential authority" or that "speak for the agent".

Whereas the targets of the analyses have been picked out by different terms, philosophers have often—although not invariably—employed the notion of identification as an element of the analysis. I have argued here that it is important to distinguish different targets—in particular, moral responsibility and autonomy. Further, I would point out that it is easy to get mixed up, given the similarity of the language employed in the various analyses—the hierarchical framework shared by many, and the element referred to by "identification".

Despite the confusing terminology, I think we can usefully distinguish two underlying phenomena that are closely related but importantly different. Understood in terms of identification, the two kinds of phenomena are structurally similar in that they essentially involve uniting different parts of the self, so to speak; that is, they both involve bringing together different elements of the mind or perhaps connecting one's action to certain elements of the mind.

On this sort of picture, when one acts in such a way as to be morally responsible, one identifies with one's action in the sense that one chooses and acts in accordance with a certain mental element or structure—the element or structure that specifies moral-responsibility identification. On Frankfurt's 1971 view, this element or structure is a second-order volition. And when one acts autonomously, one also identifies with one's action; but here one chooses and acts in accordance with a different mental element or structure—the element or structure that specifies autonomy-identification. These items (relevant to autonomy) may be a set of aims or goals specified by one's theory of autonomy, or they may be set of judgments based on value (on Watson's approach).

So acting freely in the sense relevant to moral responsibility and acting freely in the sense relevant to autonomy are structurally parallel; they both involve linking specified elements with one's choices and/or behavior. But the elements in question may well be different. On Frankfurt's 1971 view, the highlighted element related to moral responsibility is a second-order volition. In his later work, the specified aims and goals are ones the agent *cares* about or *loves*. These are interpreted in part in terms of second-order volitions, but Frankfurt adds elements to the analysis, which suggests autonomy-identification. Also, the aims and goals relevant to Taylor's view of autonomy require a certain sort of reflection involving strong evaluation, and the relevant elements in Watson's view somehow stem from "reason" or reflection on value. In general, then, there is both a structural similarity between moral responsibility and autonomy at an abstract level and an important difference: the mental elements with which choice and action are to be linked are more "robust" in the case of autonomy than moral responsibility.

Given the similarities between the two notions, and the similar analytical frameworks and terminology employed in them, it is perhaps easy to conflate the two separate ideas. But it is important to keep them separate. In particular, it might well turn out that analyses that are inadequate to give an account of autonomy are quite promising with respect to moral responsibility. In seeking to understand what moral responsibility is, it is crucial to remember what moral responsibility is not.[18]

## References


Bransen. 1996, January. Identification and the Idea of An Alternative of Oneself. *European Journal of Philosophy* 4: 1–16.

———. 2000, January. Alternatives of Oneself: Recasting Some of Our Practical Problems. *Philosophy and Phenomenological Research* 60: 381–400.

Bratman, Michael. 2003. A Desire of One's Own. *Journal of Philosophy* 100: 221–242; reprinted in Bratman 2007, 137–161.

———. 2007. *Structures of Agency*. New York: Oxford University Press.

Eshleman, Andrew. 2004. Responsibility for Character. *Philosophical Topics* 32: 65–94.

Fischer, John M. 2002. Frankfurt-Style Compatibilism. In *Contours of Agency: Essays on Themes from Harry Frankfurt*, ed. S. Buss and L. Overton, 1–26. Cambridge, MA: MIT Press.

———. 2006. *My Way: Essays on Moral Responsibility*. New York: Oxford University Press.

———. 2010. Responsibility and Autonomy. In *A Companion to the Philosophy of Action*, ed. T. O'Connor and C. Sandis, 309–316. Oxford: Wiley/Blackwell.


[18] I have benefitted from very helpful comments on previous versions of this paper by Justin Coates and Benjamin Mitchell-Yellin. Also, I delivered the paper at the conference on "Thick (Concepts of) Autonomy" at the University of Münster in October, 2012, and I am especially grateful to helpful discussions on that occasion with Michael Quante, Alfred Mele, James Taylor, and John Christman.

———. 2012. Responsibility and Autonomy: The Problem of Mission Creep. *Philosophical Issues* 22, Action Theory: 165–184.
Frankfurt, Harry G. 1969. Alternate Possibilities and Moral Responsibility. *Journal of Philosophy* 66: 829–839.
———. 1971. Freedom of the Will and the Concept of a Person. *Journal of Philosophy* 68: 5–20.
———. 1976. Identification and Externality. In *The Identities of Person*, ed. A.O. Rorty, 239–251. Berkeley: University of California Press.
———. 1982. The Importance of What We Care About. *Synthese* 53: 252–272.
———. 1987. Identification and Wholeheartedness. In *Responsibility, Character, and Emotions*, ed. F.D. Shoeman, 27–45. Cambridge: Cambridge University Press; reprinted in *Perspectives on Moral Responsibility*, eds. J. M. Fischer and M. Ravizza, 170–187. 1993. Ithaca: Cornell University Press.
———. 1988. *The Importance of What We Care About*. Cambridge: Cambridge University Press.
———. 1999a. On Caring: I. Caring and Necessity. In *Necessity, Volition, and Love, delivered as part of the Kant Lectures at Stanford University*, 155–166. Cambridge: Cambridge University Press.
———. 1999b. On Caring: II. The Necessities of Love. In *Necessity, Volition, and Love, delivered as part of the Kant Lectures at Stanford University*, 167–180. Cambridge: Cambridge University Press.
———. 2002. Reply to John Martin Fischer ["Frankfurt-Style Compatibilism"]. In *Contours of Agency: Essays on Themes from Harry Frankfurt*, ed. S. Buss and L. Overton, 27–31. Cambridge, MA: MIT Press.
———. 2004. *The Reasons of Love*. Princeton/Oxford: Princeton University Press.
———. 2006. In *Taking Ourselves Seriously and Getting It Right*, The Tanner Lectures in Moral Philosophy, ed. D. Satz. Stanford: Stanford University Press.
Mitchell-Yellin, Benjamin. 2012. *Self-Governance, Moral Responsibility, and Weakness of the Will: In Defense of the Platonic Model*. PhD Dissertation, Department of Philosophy, University of California, Riverside.
Taylor, Charles. 1976. Responsibility for Self. In *The Identities of Persons*, ed. A.O. Rorty, 281–299. Berkeley: University of California Press.
Velleman, J. David. 1992. What Happens When Someone Acts? *Mind* 101: 461–481; reprinted in *Perspectives on Moral Responsibility*, eds. J. M. Fischer and M. Ravizza, 188–210. 1993. Ithaca: Cornell University Press.
Watson, Gary. 1975. Free Agency. *Journal of Philosophy* 72: 205–220; reprinted in *Moral Responsibility*, ed. J. M. Fischer, 81–96. 1986. Ithaca: Cornell University Press.
———. 1977. Skepticism About Weakness of the Will. *Philosophical Review* 86: 316–339.
———. 1987. Free Action and Free Will. *Mind* 96: 145–172.
———. 1999. Disordered Appetites. In *Addiction: Entries and Exits*, ed. J. Elster, 3–28. New York: Russell Sage Publications.
———. 2003. The Work of the Will. In *Weakness of Will and Practical Irrationality*, ed. S. Stroud and C. Tappolet, 172–200. Oxford: Oxford University Press.
Wikipedia. 2011. *Mission Creep*. Last modified April 29, 2020. http://en.wikipedia.org/wiki/Mission_creepm. Accessed 1 June 2011.

# Chapter 2
# The Passivity of Self-Satisfaction: A Critical Re-appraisal of Harry Frankfurt's Normatively Thin Ontology of Autonomy

**Joel Anderson**

**Abstract** This chapter attempts to "re-boot" the discussion of Harry Frankfurt's approach to autonomy, in the service of a new diagnosis of the strengths and weaknesses of his satisfaction-based ontology of the will. Criticisms of Frankfurt's work have tended to focus on a lack of normative foundations, often missing Frankfurt's aim of shifting discussions of autonomy towards a focus on avoiding passivity in how one cares about what one cares about, while still acknowledging the central role of volitional necessity and, especially, self-satisfaction in autonomous agency. Although this approach provides Frankfurt with interesting ways of deflecting criticisms that are ethical in character, the lack of attention to the hermeneutic and linguistic dimensions of our inner life, leaves his approach with insufficient grounds for identifying the passivity of those who are unable or unwilling to engage in genuine self-interpretation.

## 2.1 Re-booting the Debate Over Second-Order Desires

There is a familiar depiction of the development of Harry Frankfurt's approach to autonomy that goes something like this. Frankfurt started out arguing that one is autonomous only if one has reflected critically on one's desires and figured out which desires one really wants to have. But then it was pointed out that these "second-order desires" of self-assessment are themselves mere desires, and thus also in need of further assessment – "third-order desires" – and a regress of justification ensues. According to the standard story, Frankfurt struggled with this regress problem and then ended up settling for a normatively anemic view, according to which all that matters is the coherence and harmony within the will. This turn to

J. Anderson (✉)
Utrecht University, Utrecht, The Netherlands
e-mail: j.h.Anderson@uu.nl



J. F. Childress, M. Quante (eds.), *Thick (Concepts of) Autonomy*, Philosophical Studies Series 146, https://doi.org/10.1007/978-3-030-80991-1_2

wholeheartedness, it is then often argued, is often thought of as deeply problematic. Some view too strong a requirement, in the sense that it seems to rule out a variety of perfectly acceptable forms of ambivalence. For others, the problem is that it is not strongly critical enough, in that it is value-neutral approach that can't rule out the possibility that one might be wholeheartedly evil.[1]

Unfortunately, this way of framing the discussion of the approach misses much of Frankfurt's originality, and he has spent much of the last 40 years trying to make clear that his aim is not to defend a moral theory of the person or of autonomy. However rich his account of the person and the will, it is intended to be normatively thin. With regard to the "regress objection," Frankfurt made the point himself already in 1976. As he put it later, "The mere fact that one desire occupies a higher level than another in the hierarchy seems plainly insufficient to endow it with greater authority or with any constitutive legitimacy" (Frankfurt 1988d, 166–7).[2] Clearly, the view he has been promoting in not simply one of a nested hierarchy of attitudes.

Moreover, the moralistic objections to Frankfurt's approach similarly miss their target. I recall Frankfurt saying, in a discussion after delivering a paper ("The Faintest Passion") at Northwestern University in 1992, that he is not making claims about morality but about "the ontology of the will" and that, from that perspective, there is no reason to expect wholeheartedness to serve as a moral criterion. As he put it then, "Stormtroopers can be wholehearted." Or, as he puts it more recently, "Being wholehearted is quite compatible….with being dreadfully and irredeemably wicked" (Frankfurt 2004, 98). For many, this is rather too thin, in terms of normativity. For Frankfurt, this neutrality regarding the autonomous will is not a bug; it's a feature.

In light of these misunderstandings, then, it is time for what Hollywood calls a "re-boot".[3] It's time to go back to the core motivating problem that Frankfurt is concerned with, to reconsider his proposed solution to the problem that he is actually addressing, and then – but only then – to point out where it runs aground. The point is not to search through the archives of the early work of Frankfurt, but to take a fresh look at the core ideas, without the obsession with the regress problem.

[1] The concern with moral rectitude and the regress of justification is was central to early discussions of Frankfurt's position, including (Benson 1987), (Christman 1991), (Friedman 1986), (Watson 1975), and the more recent (Wolf 2002).

[2] This is already clear in the 1976 essay, (Frankfurt 1988c, 58–68, esp. pp.65–6).

[3] The concept of a "re-boot" is used to describe a recent trend in comic books and film or TV series, in which goes back to the beginning of a serial development and makes a fresh start. See http://en.wikipedia.org/wiki/Reboot_(fiction)

## 2.2 The Problem Our Desires Pose

One of the fascinating things about animals and very young children is that they are not troubled by their desires. There is an appealing purity to the way in which they pursue what they want. They may strategize about how best to realize their goals or adjust their plans when these efforts are frustrated. But they don't worry about their desires or question their goals.

This is not a purity that is available to us as persons. It is a defining, constitutive characteristic of persons that we can and do ask ourselves whether our desires, urges, cravings, etc. deserve to be heeded. Often we don't stop to think about our desires, and often we are perfectly happy with the desires we have. But not only is it the case that we can and do question our desires, it is something that we expect of one another. It is on these grounds that Frankfurt famously distinguishes "persons" from what he calls "wantons," creatures who don't really care what they desire (Frankfurt 1988b). His central idea is that the capacity to be troubled by these conflicts is a necessary feature of the ontology of the will of persons.

There is admittedly something distasteful about the whole business of dividing "genuine persons" from "mere wantons", animals, or whatever. We can easily get wrapped up in debates about what the best terms are here, or about what makes a creature "really human". But I think Frankfurt is correct to say that there is a fundamental watershed that exists between those creatures who ask the question of whether their desires are undesirable and those who don't. In what follows, I will continue to refer to the first set of creatures by employing the technical philosophical term, "we".

For us, then, desires (like beliefs) can and do pose questions. Frankfurt recently put this in a particularly stark fashion:

> [T]he mere fact that a person has a desire does not give him a reason. *What it gives him is a problem.* He has the problem of whether to identify with the desire and thus validate it as eligible for satisfaction, or whether to dissociate himself from it, treat it as categorically unacceptable, and try to suppress it or rid himself of it entirely (Frankfurt 2006: 11, emphasis added).

Our desires raise issues that we must resolve. But the option of solving the problem by simply treating all our desires as automatically reasons is not an option that is available to us – not to anyone who is still one of us. There is no way back. We must move forward. Call this "the predicament of volitional reflexivity."

The predicament of volitional reflexivity is a bit like the Garden of Eden after the Fall. Having eaten from the tree of critical self-knowledge, our situation is transformed, and we must find a way to move forward. Seen this way, Frankfurt's philosophical work is, at a most fundamental level, about the question of what it means to handle this predicament in a mature way. Whether one refers to it as "maturity", "genuine personhood," "the highest good," "freedom of the will," or "autonomy," the primary normative goal of Frankfurt's writings is to develop an account of what can count as a successful response to the predicament of volitional reflexivity – a predicament that emerges from the internal structure of the will.

Implicit in Frankfurt's writings is the claim that the predicament is a general phenomenon, part of the human condition. But it presents itself in specific cases. Suppose you find yourself increasingly drawn to play a more active role in politics. Suppose, in particular, that you find yourself with a strong desire to run for local political office. The predicament is that you have to figure out what to do with this desire. Do you really stand behind this desire, or is it a distraction from what you really care about, something that snuck up on you via a flattering remark from a neighbor or a wave of panic about a current political crisis? Engaging with these questions – "taking ourselves seriously" as Frankfurt puts it in the title of his Tanner Lectures – involves taking a stand with regard to one's will and facing the predicament squarely.

## 2.3 Passive Failures to Face the Predicament of Volitional Reflexivity

Before continuing, it is important to get clear on what is so problematic about failing to face the predicament. Why should we let our desires bother us? For Frankfurt, the answer lies in understanding how such refusals represent the *passivity* that characterizes non-persons (or "wantons").

The most extreme form of passivity is not to care at all what desires one has and what one's will is like. As we saw earlier, this degree of passivity puts one under the threshold of full personhood, on Frankfurt's account. There are interesting debates to be had here, about the nature of personhood, but my concern here is with cases in which we are passive about inner conflicts, cases in which there is a real danger of remaining a mere spectator to the inner struggles between our desires.[4] Take the example of someone who has a strong desire to retaliate when slighted. Suppose he receives an email circulated to his department at work, in which it is suggested that he was responsible for a situation in which the entire department was embarrassed. Suppose this gives rise, as it so often does, to two competing inclinations: to lash out with counter-accusations in an email CC'ed to the entire department, or to demonstrate to his skeptical colleagues that he is, in fact, capable of acting like a grownup. To be passive here is not really care how this internal conflict plays out. It is, in that sense, to be a bystander.

It is important to emphasize that overcoming passivity, in Frankfurt's sense, does not guarantee that the rejected desire will *disappear* or cease to both one (Frankfurt 1988d, 175). Rather, when we take an active stand regarding which side of the conflict we want to win – in Frankfurt's language, when we "identify" with one side – we make it the case that the failure of that desire to win the conflict would be felt as

[4] It is worth noting that Frankfurt here departs from much of contemporary empirical psychology, as well as the work of philosophers such as Daniel Dennett, builds on the idea that we are, in fact, bystanders to the process in which action is generated as the result of a competition between different subpersonal agents (e.g., Dennett 2003).

a loss. The conflict is not thereby terminated, but its character is fundamentally altered. Frankfurt's way of putting this is to say that the conflict ceases to be a conflict within oneself. For the conflict can now be described as being one between "...what the person really wants and other desires...that are *external* to the volitional complex with which the person identifies and by which he wants his behavior to be determined" (Frankfurt 1988d, 165). What this means is that although one is no longer torn or divided or confused about what one wants, one may still find oneself continuing to have both of the conflicting desires. It is thus not Frankfurt's claim that the wholehearted person has no internal conflicts. The desire to send the spiteful email may continue to pester and fester. In wholeheartedly rejecting one desire and endorsing the other, what one resolves is not the conflict but oneself (Frankfurt 1988d, 100; Frankfurt 1998b, 164).

Often, however, we struggle with which stand to take, and these uncertainties raise deeper or higher-order questions with regard to which we must also take a stand. And here, too, like bystanders who unsure of how to respond to a crime in progress, we can end up rendered passive by our volitional incoherence.

In Frankfurt's writings, one can distinguish between two ways in which volitional incoherence can threaten the self. On the one hand, there is *ambivalence*, in which one is torn between committing oneself and not committing oneself to a given person, project, or ideal; on the other hand, there is the paralyzing *disorientation* of being pulled in so many different directions that one does not know what one wants. Both forms of volitional incoherence undermine one's autonomy, but in different ways.

Ambivalence is a matter of one's being at cross-purposes at the highest level of one's reflective endorsements (Frankfurt 1988d; Frankfurt 1998b; Frankfurt 2004; for a discussion, see (Swindell 2010) and (Velleman 2002)).

For example, someone considering running for political office could be deeply and authentically committed to improving society and, equally, to sparing his family the added strains of his taking on extra responsibilities, but circumstances make these two commitments incompatible. In cases of ambivalence, the agent is seriously divided with regard to this internal conflict. Frankfurt describes the phenomenon this way:

> The disunity of an ambivalent person's will prevents him from effectively pursuing and satisfactorily attaining his goals. Like conflict within reason, volitional conflict leads to self-betrayal and self-defeat. The trouble is in each case the same: a sort of incoherent greed – trying to have things both ways – which naturally makes it impossible to get anywhere. The flow of volitional or of intellectual activity is interrupted and reversed; movement in any direction is truncated and turned back. However a person starts out how to decide or to think, he finds that he is getting in his own way (Frankfurt 1998b, 99).

Frankfurt not denying here, I take it, that it may be essential for psychological health to be able to acknowledge conflicting feelings or to grieve the losses incurred even in making the right decision.[5] The point is simply that, if we are to move forward,

[5] Here I am in agreement with critics such as Rössler (Rössler 2009) who argue that Frankfurt's concept of 'wholeheartedness' is incompatible with this sort of awareness of mixed feelings. In

we must not be passive bystanders but must face up to the predicament of being aware of the incoherencies in our will.

There is also a second form of volitional incoherence about which one might be passive, something we could call "disorientation". Whereas the phenomenology of ambivalence is one of being pulled in two directions, the feeling associated with disorientation is of being aimless. Frequently, according to Frankfurt, this is the result of having more options and few constraints:

> …[Someone with more options] may become, to a greater or lesser degree, disoriented with respect to where his interests and preferences lie. Instead of finding that the scope and vigor of his autonomy are augmented as the ranges of choices open to him broadens, he may become volitionally debilitated by an increasing uncertainty both concerning how to make decisions and concerning what to choose (Frankfurt 1998a, 109; see also Frankfurt 1998b, 101–03; Dworkin 1988).

Disorientation involves a lack of "flow" and vigor, which leaves one feeling frustrated or just apathetic, but also usually means that one, here again, gets in one's own way. These negative characteristics add to the rhetorical force of Frankfurt's discussion, but the core argument I believe is again one about passivity. The problem is not that one lacks some objectively good degree of integration but that one is negligently passive about the fact that one's volitional makeup leaves one incapable of resolving the conflict effectively. Seen this way, I think it is a mistake to interpret Frankfurt as obsessed with volitional coherence. His reasoning is ultimately rather instrumental: the threat posed by disorientation (and other forms of volitional incoherence) lies in the way it leaves one unable to resolve conflicts. Failure to figure out where one stands thus involves, indirectly, negligent passivity with regard to internal conflicts, since we need to know where to stand to know how to resolve them. And it passivity about internal conflicts, I am arguing, that constitutes the basis of Frankfurt's implicit claims about the structure of a good will.

Ambivalence and disorientation both represent, then, forms of volitional incoherence that undermine a person's active, purposeful agency. Frankfurt's way of making his point is typically in terms the phenomenology of its opposite: we feel most freely self-directing, he suggests, when our minds are made up, when we are so decisively resolved to follow a certain course of action that nothing distracts us from the flow of our activity. In this sense, making up one's mind has a *liberating* effect (Frankfurt 1988e, 88; Frankfurt 1998a, 110). But his claim has less to do with how one experiences oneself than with the objective character of one's will. When we take a stand, we may still be engaged in a struggle with desires, temptations, and so, but we are no longer passive bystanders.

---

response to a similar objection from David Velleman, Frankfurt writes: "Resolving ambivalence by taking a decisive stand against certain feelings does not require (or even permit) that a person misrepresent those feelings or that he conceal them from himself" (Frankurt 2002c, 126).

## 2.4 Facing the Predicament and Resolving One's Will: Structural Hierarchicalism of the Will

In general, then, Frankfurt's position is that one can avoid being a passive bystander towards one's desires and, more broadly, towards the health of one's will by taking a stand with regard to one's will. By itself, this can sound rather arbitrary, and indeed, there was a decisionistic strain in Frankfurt's early claim that what one needs most in identifying with or rejecting one's desires is to do so *decisively* (Frankfurt 1988b, 21). Since a position like that is unable to rule out cases of people being decisive from moment to moment, and yet flip-flopping and vacillating constantly over time, Frankfurt has moved towards a position that emphasizes the ways in which the structure of one's will anchors one's actions, feelings, responses, and so on.

As I noted at the outset, however, having the right structure, for Frankfurt, is not a matter of tracking some independent reality of a true self or even of moral values. His normatively thin approach centers on structural features of the will. He frequently uses the term "wholeheartedness" for the requisite state of the will, in which one responds effectively to the predicament of volitional reflexivity. But my sense is that what has emerged most recently as his preferred language for talking about this is the language of "satisfaction" with oneself. Since self-satisfaction is rarely treated as the hallmark of a mature, autonomous person, this requires some explanation.

What we are looking for, according to Frankfurt, is a state of the will in which one has actively taken a stand on the inclinations one finds oneself with, but where this stand is not arbitrary or fickle or otherwise inherently unstable. This is the ideal towards which persons strive when they respond to predicaments. It is, in his view, the only way to resolve the predicament with which choice presents us.

Avoiding arbitrariness requires that one's identification with a desire be accompanied by a certain degree of integration and equilibrium within the volitional makeup of the person, and the term "satisfaction" is actually not such a strange choice here:

> Hierarchical accounts of the identity of the self do not presume, however, that a person's identification with some desire consists simply in the fact that he *has* a higher-order desire by which the first desire is endorsed. The endorsing higher-order desire must be, in addition, a desire with which the person is *satisfied* (Frankfurt 1998b, 105).

The central requirement of this condition of satisfaction is that one be free from uneasiness about this identification, that one have no particular inclination to reconsider the identification. Being satisfied with endorsing a desire to perform a particular action is compatible with the counterfactual claim that, had one endorsed a desire not to perform that action, one would have been satisfied with that (Frankfurt 1998b, 103–04). Crucial to this argument is the further claim that not going to a yet-higher level of reflection is not a matter of *refusing* to do so. As a deliberate act or decision, such a refusal would be open to the suspicion that it might be motivated by a desire that one would not endorse, and trying to establish the authority or wholeheartedness of this refusal itself would spawn an endless series of further reflections. But one might also simply be *satisfied* with one's identification with a given first-order desire. And this, Frankfurt argues, avoids the problem entirely:

> Satisfaction with one's self requires, then, no adoption of any cognitive, attitudinal, affective, or intentional stance. It does not require the performance of a particular act; and it also does not require any deliberate abstention. Satisfaction is a state of the entire psychic system – a state constituted just by the absence of any tendency or inclination to alter its condition" (Frankfurt 1998b, 104).

More recently, has articulated his position regarding self-satisfaction, in connection with Spinoza's claim that the highest good is "*acquiescentia in se ipso.*" (Frankfurt 2006, 17). In answer to the question, why "acquiescing to oneself" is the *highest* thing one can hope for, Frankfurt says this:

> Perhaps because it resolves the deepest problem. In our transition beyond naïve animality, we separate from ourselves and disrupt our original unreflective spontaneity. This puts us at risk to varieties of inner fragmentation, dissonance, and disorder. Accepting ourselves reestablishes the wholeness that was undermined by our elementary constitutive maneuvers of division and distancing. When we are acquiescent to ourselves, or willing freely, there is no conflict within the structure of our motivations and desires. We have successfully negotiated our distinctively human complexity. The unity of our self has been restored (Frankfurt 2006, 18).

This, it seems to me, is as close to a definitive statement of Frankfurt core position as one can find in any of his writings. There is the idea of what I am calling the "predicament," which is clearly part of the human condition. It is resolved at a level that is both volitional and, as he puts it in the next sentence, "purely structural". And there is the equation of "willing freely" with not being internally divided. Self-satisfaction and self-acceptance thus represent a mature way of facing the predicament that our desires pose.

## 2.5 How Critical Must Volitional Reflexivity Be?

At this point the key question arises regarding the implications of this normatively thin ontology of the will: is it not possible that people are too easily satisfied with themselves? Isn't this the ultimate form of passivity? What ever happened to the idea that autonomous agency is a matter of reflecting *critically* on one's first-order desires?

In a way, however, this line of objection misunderstands Frankfurt's project. As I have been emphasizing throughout, what he is offering is an account of how we can successfully respond to the predicament that arises from our natural inclination to be critical. Self-critical doubt is thus the *problem* to be solved, and the question for Frankfurt is how one can solve it while still being a person who actively cares about his will.

The notion of self-satisfaction actually captures the approach quite well. As Frankfurt argues, "Being satisfied with the way things are is unmistakably an excellent reason for having no great interest in changing them" (Frankfurt 1988a, 155). It is, moreover, a normatively thin and value-neutral reason, based on a formal, structural ontology of the will of persons. Thus, in a situation in which one is genuinely settled on what one cares about, desires, and loves, one has successfully faced the questions raised by having those cares, desires, and loves. In that regard, more critical reflection contributes nothing further. Despite his emphasis on the capacity for reflection as a condition for personhood, Frankfurt is deeply concerned with the way in which demands for critical reflection can run amok and end up blocking individuals' capacity ever to resolve to do anything.

This is where it becomes clear that the ideal of mature agency that Frankfurt aims to capture with "self-satisfaction" is closely tied to the notion of confidence. Indeed, he concludes his Tanner Lectures with the claim that it is confidence – rather than, one might add, intersubjective confirmation – that "provides us with the deepest and most secure foundation for practical reason" (Frankfurt 2006, 52). But this is an old theme for Frankfurt. In the spirit of a "re-boot," it is worth recalling Frankfurt's origin story as a Descartes scholar and the interpretation of Cartesian epistemological foundations in terms of a feeling of confidence:

> Descartes cares less about the correspondence of his beliefs to "reality" than he does about their permanence and constancy. What he wishes above all to avoid is not error, in the sense of non-correspondence, but betrayal. What might be *found out* to be false is what he wishes to guard against. If a belief can confidently be expected to remain unshaken by any further inquiry, that is all the truth he cares to demand" (Frankfurt 1970, 180).[6]

At this point, a critic could challenge Frankfurt on the cogency of grounding epistemic warrant in a feeling of confidence. Indeed, I have done so elsewhere (Anderson 2003). Given the prevalence of *over* confidence, after all, felt confidence would appear to provide appropriate grounding for judgments on how to live only when it is *warranted* confidence. Ultimately, I think that following this question (as to the justification for trusting our feelings of confidence) will reveal the limits of a purely subjective and individualistic approach such as Frankfurt's. Without public criteria or procedures that transcend subjective consciousness, it is impossible to make a principled distinction between what seems to be justified and what is justified.

But this is not the line of criticism that I wish to pursue here. Instead, I want to identify a different sort of dissatisfaction that I have with Frankfurt's way of framing the predicament of volitional reflexivity.

[6] See also Frankfurt, (Frankfurt 1988d, 169), where Frankfurt mentions that his understanding of unreserved commitment or identification "owes much to Descartes's discussion of clear and distinct perception." For a fuller discussion, see (Anderson 1996, ch. 3.2), and (Herman 2002, 259), together with Frankfurt's reply (Frankurt 2002a, 275–78).

## 2.6 Self-Opacity and the Importance of Understanding What We Care About

Suppose I can respond confidently to a predicament of volitional reflexivity. The "problem" posed by my desires is resolved wholeheartedly by my taking a stand on whether I identify with or reject these desires. I could, in principle, continue to probe whether I *really* care about what I think I care about, but if I am satisfied with where I stand, it's not clear what the point of doing that would be. My life may not work out as I hope, but at least I can get on with it.

That, then, is Frankfurt's basic picture of a mature and healthy will, and as I have suggested throughout, it is not easily dismissed. Nevertheless, I do believe that there is something missing. The problem, in short, is that Frankfurt overlooks the extent to which resolving the problem of volitional reflexivity involves *making sense* of the position one takes. For someone might be wholeheartedly and confident and yet not really understand her desires. One might be satisfied with oneself but opaque to oneself. To illustrate the sort of wholehearted self-opacity that I have in mind, consider the following case, from a National Public Radio profile of the late Rev. Robert Shields of Dayton, Washington (Isay 1994, accessible at https://storycorps.org/stories/worlds-longest-diary/).

From 1972 to 1997, Shields kept an extraordinarily meticulous diary, typing up the minute-by-minute occurrences in his life. It totalled 37.5 million words, and the detail is overwhelming. At periodic intervals during the day, Shields recorded how many ounces of juice he drank at breakfast, what the morning newspaper weighed, what he read, when he went to the bathroom, what the barometer reading was, and how much time he spent speed-typing his journal. Even in retirement, his journal kept him very busy. Indeed, the diary usually took up so much time that he had no time to read it – and apparently little interest in doing so. In the radio interview, there is a rushed tone to his voice, as he keeps typing rather than taking time to answer the interviewer's questions. At one point in that interview, the following exchange occurs:

> Isay: "Why are you doing this?…What are you trying to do?"
>
> Shields: "I don't know. I don't really – I really can't answer that. [He reads the text aloud as he continues typing] Five-forty-five to 6:15 I read more from the Oxford Dictionary of Quotations. I ate half a dozen large Archway sugar cookies while I drank two cups of milk." …..
>
> Isay: "How does your family feel about this?"
>
> Shields: "Never asked them." [laughs]
>
> Isay: "What about leaving town?"
>
> Shields: "I don't leave town. I haven't left town since 1985, to visit my brother in Tennessee. I don't like to be away overnight because it gets me behind. If I travel to Walla Walla to do shopping, it puts me behind in the diary. I have to take notes all the time, and…it takes almost a day to catch up with the notes. So I avoid going out. I avoid being away. [He begins typing again.] Three-O-five to 3:30, I read the *Tri-City Herald*…."

In terms of Frankfurt's criteria, Rev. Shields is a model of wholehearted caring. He explicitly endorsed his desire to continue with the diary. And he obviously *cared* about it. Indeed, he had a half-dozen typewriters set up to guard against the loss that would otherwise threaten were one of the them to break down. And his aversion to leaving town is grounded in the fact that he did not want to betray his project or himself.

Yet Rev. Shields had very little idea why he was doing what he was doing, and this is the point of the example for my purposes. When pressed, during the interview, to explain why he keeps the diary, he draws a blank. He does not really understand his own actions. He is unable to provide even a minimally plausible account of what he is up to, incapable of rendering his way of life – and the choices that reproduce it – intelligible. Although it is possible that he was just shy, he appears to have been unable to make sense of his life, even to *himself*. And then it is hard to see how he wasn't somehow failing to face fully the predicament of volitional reflexivity. His failure to make sense of himself illustrates yet another form of passivity.

At this point, in the concluding two sections, I would like to take up two ways in which Frankfurt could respond to the charge that his account overlooks the importance of understanding oneself. One response is to say that intelligibility *does* matter, but that those who are wholehearted have all the intelligibility that is required for active personhood. Alternatively, one can deny that the predicament of volitional reflexivity requires intelligibility at all. In the remainder of this essay, I will try to say briefly where I think that both of these responses run aground.

## 2.7 Frankfurt's Hermeneutically Impoverished Ontology of the Will

The first response would be for Frankfurt to argue that there is something like "*volitional* intelligibility" and that this is sufficient for an agent to count as being able to make sense of his responses. To develop this line of argument, one could start with David Velleman's discussion of intelligibility as a necessary condition for action. After all, we continue acting only if we understand what we are going to do. If, to use his example, you are walking up Fifth Avenue and you suddenly realize you don't know where you are going, this pulls you up short (Velleman 1989, 15–17). In Frankfurt's language, you don't know where you stand with regard to where you want to go. Building on this idea, one could defend Frankfurt's approach by saying that he has a *volitional* understanding of "intelligibility." As Frankfurt says in another context, "the fact that someone cares about something, or that something is important to him, means just that the person is disposed to behave in certain ways" (Frankurt 2002b, 161). What we get, then, is an account of what it means for our actions to "make sense" to us that is cashed out in terms of its covariance with a confident, wholehearted exercise of the will. In this sense, it is sufficient evidence for Rev. Shields's diary project being intelligible to him that he pursued it wholeheartedly, which he most certainly did. As Frankfurt would likely say, if he was fully satisfied with his caring, it's unclear what more he could have reasonably needed in the way of evidence for thinking that it *made sense* for him to care.

In effect, however, this response involves answering the objection by deflating the notion of "intelligibility" beyond recognition. After all, the starting intuition of the objection was that someone like Rev. Shields might be perfectly wholehearted but lack any way of fitting his commitments into a larger context in which it makes sense. Mere behavior cannot provide sense of "fitting in", because bodily movements by themselves make no reference to a larger constellation of meaning. The interesting question is whether this sense of fitting in can be provided by the reflexivity of the will central to Frankfurt's account, according to which caring about something entails, for example, a commitment to ensuring that one's will is so structured that one continues to care. But here Frankfurt seems to face a dilemma. On the one hand, he could stick to the largely dispositional account, in which case he has to deny any necessary role for the inferential links between possible courses of action. Seen this way, Rev. Shields would count as "understanding" what he was up to, even though he had nothing to say about how the various things he cared about fit together. On the other hand, Frankfurt could allow that caring involves a sensitivity to these inferential connections, such that Shields's caring about updating his diary needs to fit with his response to specific situations as well as his caring about other connections. Frankfurt could indeed argue that, as a matter of fact, we won't be satisfied, confident, and wholehearted if we aren't on the attuned to the discordance between different things we care about. Seen in this way, Frankfurt could say that his theory does not actually force him to deny that there are problems with the Rev. Shields's volitional coherence, for Shields may have been rigidly cutting himself off from dimensions of his caring and thus revealing himself to be a "wanton" with regard to those dimensions. That said, it's entirely unclear how this emphasis on self-understanding, much as I would welcome it, is something that Frankfurt could integrate into this theory. For I see no way of developing such an approach without making judgment and reasons-responsiveness a central part of a richer conception (and thus requirement) of self-understanding. In other words, what is needed is a thicker conception of the forms of hermeneutic agency that are necessary for being able to make sense of even our most mundane commitments. And that is something that Frankfurt has consistently viewed as unnecessary to a healthy, mature, confident will.

## 2.8 The Costs of Frankfurt's Commitments to Thinness

Alternatively, Frankfurt could defend his normatively thin ontology of the will by rejecting the requirement of intelligibility. However important intelligibility might be to some people, he could argue, it is not necessary for the kind of volitional coherence that concerns us here. It is, thus, an *optional* part of a mature response to the predicament of volitional reflexivity – and perhaps a part that reflects a particular, substantive value-commitment on the part of members of cultural elites. On a parallel with Frankfurt's separation of questions of ethics from questions of caring, one could say that, if you care about having a deep and articulate understanding of your motives, that's fine; it may help you win friends and influence people; but it would be a mistake to see self-understanding and wholeheartedness as linked in any essential way.

That is, I think, the most consistent position for Frankfurt to take, since it fits with his general suspicions regarding the normative overburdening of concepts employed in discussions of how to lead one's life. Frankfurt effectively and repeatedly puts the burden of proof on those who would say that personhood, autonomy, genuine caring, or what have you somehow requires "more". And, while I can appreciate the wisdom of his caution against an endless pursuit of "the better" at the cost of "the good," I believe that his culture-critic's aversion to spoiled adults with limitless expectations (Frankfurt 1982, 319) has distracted him from the importance of avoiding the form of passivity involved is acquiescing to self-opacity, to not understanding oneself.

The passivity I have in mind is a form of disregard that comes into view when one takes a broader view of the way in which our inner life engages us when we reflect. Frankfurt operates on the assumption that the mode in which desires present themselves as requiring a response is the mode of a problem that calls for volitional resolution. In this sense, the predicament of reflexivity we face as persons is to be seen in terms of problems to be solved, in the way a pain in one's back calls for adjusting how one sits. But there is actually a much wider range of ways in which our inner life calls for a response. Indeed, part of what is distinctive about the predicament of volitional reflexivity that we face is this. We find our desires, emotions, aversions, and so on not just troubling and unsettling but *perplexing*. It is not merely *problems* that our desires pose; they also pose *questions*.[7] And the grammar of answering questions adequately is different from that of resolving problems adequately. In particular, the success conditions are different. We know when volitional problems are resolved; we can feel it. But questions are more complex, and, although there are better answers and worse answers, there is in principle always more to say.

This, it seems to me, is why Frankfurt's model of mature, confident, wholehearted self-satisfaction is – despite its nuance, elegance, and prudence – ultimately rather unsatisfying. It fails to acknowledge the way in which our inner life presents us with ongoing, open-ended possibilities for self-interpretation, and thus with the possibility of a richer and deeper form of selfhood. We may well have reasons not to pursue all these possibilities, but Frankfurt's commitment to thinness forces him to underestimate the importance of a form of openness that is crucial to avoiding passivity. Frankfurt's satisficing emphasis on volitional stability leaves him with little to say about the form of active agency that is required for being alert to rigidity and receptive to transformation. Frankfurt has a point in warning against a

[7] This is a point that Charles Taylor has been particularly adept at expression: "We [as opposed to other animals] experience our pre-articulate emotions as perplexing, as raising a question" (Taylor 1985, 74). Regarding the complexities of the ongoing task of finding an adequate answer to the questions posed, see especially (Taylor 1989, ch. 1–4).

compulsive, constant reexamination of all one's feelings all the time, chasing after the next shiny possibility. But avoiding that extreme does not require adopting the approach that Frankfurt seems to take, in which we wait, like passive bystanders, for internal conflicts to arise. An active engagement with one's desires and opportunities, with the questions they pose, and with the perspectives of those with whom we share our lives not only fits naturally with mature and robust ontology of the will, but it may even be required for the will's dynamic character.

My diagnosis of where Frankfurt's approach comes up short here is that it neglects language and meaning (as well as experimentation and exploration) in its characterization of the predicament that arises when – often enough, because of our engagement with the world and others in it – we turn inward. We can, of course, decide to leave these issues of meaning and self-interpretation to one side. If we do so, we might well be able to live less troubled and more volitionally robust lives. But we will lack what I have elsewhere called the *hermeneutic* or *disclosive* dimension of autonomy (Anderson 2014, 149–50). We will be bystanders to these deeper, language-dependent dimensions of our lives. In refusing to engage actively with this further dimension of the predicament of volitional reflexivity, we will be, in that sense, wantons.[8]

## References

Anderson, Joel. 1996. *A Social Conception of Personal Autonomy: Volitional Identity, Strong Evaluation, and Intersubjective Accountability*. Dissertation, Northwestern University.

———. 2003. Autonomy and the Authority of Personal Commitments: From Internal Coherence to Social Normativity. *Philosophical Explorations* 6 (2): 90–108.

———. 2014. Autonomy and Vulnerability Entwined. In *Vulnerability: New Essays in Ethics and Feminist Philosophy*, ed. Catriona Mackenzie, Wendy Rogers, and Susan Dodds, 134–161. Oxford: Oxford University Press.

Benson, P. 1987. Freedom and Value. *Journal of Philosophy* 84: 465–486.

Christman, John. 1991. Autonomy and Personal History. *Canadian Journal of Philosophy* 20: 1–24.

Dennett, Daniel C. 2003. *Freedom Evolves*. New York: Viking.

Dworkin, Gerald. 1988. Is More Choice Better Than Less? In *The Theory and Practice of Autonomy*, 62–81. New York: Cambridge University Press.

Frankfurt, Harry G. 1970. *Demons, Dreamers, and Madmen: The Defense of Reason in Descartes's "Meditations"*. Indianapolis: Bobbs-Merrill.

———. 1982. Comments on Macintyre. *Synthese* 53: 319–321.

———. 1988a. Equality as a Moral Ideal. In *The Importance of What We Care About*, 134–158. New York: Cambridge University Press.

———. 1988b. Freedom of the Will and the Concept of a Person. In *The Importance of What We Care About*, 11–25. New York: Cambridge University Press.

[8] For valuable discussion and feedback, I would particularly like to thank Thomas Nys. An earlier version of this essay appeared in Dutch as "Is tevredenheid met jezelf genoeg?" in *Vrijheid, noodzaak en liefde: Een inleiding tot de filosofie van Harry Frankfurt*, ed. Katrien Schaubroeck and Thomas Nys (Kapellen: Pelckmans, 2011), pp. 75–95.)

———. 1988c. Identification and Externality. In *The Importance of What We Care About*, 58–68. New York: Cambridge University Press.

———. 1988d. Identification and Wholeheartedness. In *The Importance of What We Care About*, 159–176. New York: Cambridge University Press.

———. 1988e. *The Importance of What We Care About*. In *The Importance of What We Care About*, 80–94. New York: Cambridge University Press.

———. 1998a. *On the Necessity of Ideals*, 108–116. Cambridge: Cambridge University Press.

———. 1998b. *The Faintest Passion*, 95–107. Cambridge: Cambridge University Press.

———. 2004. *The Reasons of Love*. Princeton: Princeton University Press.

———. 2006. *Taking Ourselves Seriously and Getting it Right*. Stanford, CA: Stanford University Press.

Frankurt, Harry. 2002a. Reply to Barbara Herman. In *Contours of Agency: Essays on Themes from Harry Frankfurt*, ed. Sarah Buss and Lee Overton, 275–278. Cambridge, MA: MIT Press.

———. 2002b. Reply to Gary Watson. In *Contours of Agency: Essays on Themes from Harry Frankfurt*, ed. Sarah Buss and Lee Overton, 160–164. Cambridge, MA: MIT Press.

Frankurt, Harry G. 2002c. Reply to J. David Velleman. In *Contours of Agency: Essays on Themes from Harry Frankfurt*, ed. Sarah Buss and Lee Overton, 124–128. Cambridge, MA: MIT Press.

Friedman, Marilyn. 1986. Autonomy and the Split-Level Self. *Southern Journal of Philosophy* 24: 19–35.

Herman, Barbara. 2002. Bootstrapping. In *Contours of Agency: Essays on Themes From Harry Frankfurt*, ed. Sarah Buss and Lee Overton, 253–274. Cambridge, MA: MIT Press.

Isay, David. 1994. Robert Shields, World's Longest Diary. *Morning Edition*, National Public Radio

Rössler, Beate. 2009. Autonomie und Ambivalenz. In *Sozialphilosophie und Kritik*, ed. Rainer Forst, Martin Hartmann, Rahel Jaeggi, and Martin Saar, 359–383. Frankfurt: Suhrkamp.

Swindell, J.S. 2010. Ambivalence. *Philosophical Explorations* 13: 23–34.

Taylor, Charles. 1985. Self-Interpreting Animals. In *Human Agency and Language*, 45–76. Cambridge: Cambridge University Press.

———. 1989. *Sources of the Self: The Making of the Modern Identity*. Cambridge: Harvard University Press.

Velleman, J. David. 1989. *Practical Reflection*. Princeton: Princeton University Press.

———. 2002. Identification and Identity. In *Contours of Agency: Essays on Themes from Harry Frankfurt*, ed. Sarah Buss and Lee Overton, 91–123. Cambridge, MA: MIT Press.

Watson, Gary. 1975. Free Agency. *The Journal of Philosophy* 72 (8): 205.

Wolf, Susan. 2002. The True, the Good, and the Lovable: Frankfurt's Avoidance of Objectivity. In *Contours of Agency: Essays on Themes from Harry Frankfurt*, ed. Sarah Buss and Lee Overton, 227–244. Cambridge, MA: MIT Press.

# Chapter 3
# Determining Oneself and Determining One's Self

**Thomas Schramme**

**Abstract** In this essay, I exploit an ambiguity in the concept of self-determination. Self-de Green termination can mean to determine oneself in choices and actions or to determine one's self. The second kind of self-determination leads to our capacity to imagine alternative selves of ourselves, which are to be actualized. This creates the basis for a normative conception of self-determination, i.e. a conception that incorporates the aspect of a right or good way to determine oneself. I defend a normative interpretation of self-determination, which is illustrated by reference to three theorists: Harry Frankfurt, Thomas Hill Green and John Stuart Mill.

In this essay, I exploit an ambiguity in the concept of self-determination. Self-determination can mean to determine oneself in choices and actions or to determine one's self. I will call the first interpretation self-actualisation and the second self-formation. The second kind of self-determination leads to our capacity to imagine alternative selves of ourselves, which are to be actualized. This creates the basis for a normative conception of self-determination, i.e. a conception that incorporates the aspect of a right or good way to determine oneself. I defend a normative interpretation of self-determination, which is illustrated by reference to three theorists: Harry Frankfurt, Thomas Hill Green and John Stuart Mill.

In the first section (3.1), I set the context by describing in general terms how I conceive the connection between freedom and human beings' idea of themselves. There is a conception of self-determination that sets no limits so that any possible uncoerced way to express oneself is supposed to be self-determined. There is a second conception that introduces norms of proper forms of self-determination. I call

T. Schramme (✉)
University of Liverpool, Liverpool, UK
e-mail: t.schramme@liverpool.ac.uk



J. F. Childress, M. Quante (eds.), *Thick (Concepts of) Autonomy*, Philosophical Studies Series 146, https://doi.org/10.1007/978-3-030-80991-1_3

the former voluntarist and the second perfectionist accounts of self-determination. In the second section (3.2), I introduce the general distinction between self-actualisation and self-formation and connect them with the two accounts from section one, so that I end up with a classification of four ideal-types of theories. The following three sections discuss three versions (one is disregarded for being implausible) with historical illustrations. A version of voluntarist self-actualisation is represented by Harry Frankfurt in Sect. 3.3. In the fourth section (3.4), I discuss Thomas Hill Green's version of perfectionist self-formation, before moving on to John Stuart Mill's account of perfectionist self-actualisation in Sect. 3.5. Mill's theory seems to me the most plausible in that it allows for normative constraints of proper self-actualisation but also insists on one's own individual versions of self-determination. Section 3.6 concludes.

## 3.1 Introduction

The value of our freedom to act does not merely stem from the fact that it enables us to do things that we may, at some specific point in time, strive to do. The value of individual freedom especially derives from the desire of human beings to express themselves in the world. Human beings do not merely want to satisfy their relevant preferences, but also to realise their individual identity – the way they are – in their decisions and actions.

This necessitates a capacity to see oneself as a being that possesses and commands certain continuous attributes, such as evaluative beliefs, ideals, and a character. Restrictions to our options seem to us to be problematic wherever they bring us to do something with which we do not identify ourselves, or when we are not able to do something for which we stand. This is, in a word, the value of self-determination.

If we did not have the capacity to identify with our actions – or to distance ourselves from them – self-determination would not seem to have value to us; for whatever we would do, it would be impossible to evaluate it from our own perspective. We would simply actualise that which currently impels us to do so. If we were for instance automata, then we would not need to be concerned about whether we have actually realised ourselves or not. We would simply act, and would either be capable or incapable of doing that which is given to us as a goal, e.g. by a computer program. An automaton can have freedom to act or not, but it cannot be self-determined. Self-determination, rather, has to do with freedom of choice. Only when beings can be this or that, when they have alternative ideas of themselves arises the idea of a self and thereby the significance of whether one can realise oneself in the world or not.

The idea of self-determination is not commonly understood such that every way we express ourselves through our actions actually counts as an acceptable form of self-determination. There are indeed many examples, especially in literature and film, in which human beings do not reach their potential or "waste their lives". For instance, should we consider the life of Jeff Lebowski, also known as "The Dude", protagonist of the film *The Big Lebowski*, as a self-determined one? The Dude does not do much else than to consume drugs, to go bowling, and to take care of his shag rug.

Many philosophers believe that we human beings have a natural need to cultivate our individual capabilities as much as possible. According to this understanding of the human life the Dude would not live up to his own nature. In this manner John Rawls for instance has made the claim: "Human beings enjoy the exercise of their realized capacities (…), and this enjoyment increases the more the capacity is realized, or the greater its complexity." (Rawls 1999, 364). We could paraphrase this so-called "Aristotelian principle" of Rawls's in that human beings have a perfectible nature, and that they are interested in improving this nature. Here the connection between self-determination and happiness or the good life of human beings is clearly visible. Indeed, many would claim that only a self-determined life can be a good life. In this way it seems important *how* and *to what end* we determine ourselves.

But not to see the Dude as at all self-determined is perhaps demanding too much of a self-determined life. In the end, for all we know he has chosen his life without coercion. Is it not enough for the goal of self-determination that certain formal criteria for free choice are fulfilled? The Dude may fall short of real happiness or he may simply foster some sort of unconventional interpretation of the good life, but he lives his life in self-determined fashion all the same. From this point of view there would be no prescribed external norms of proper self-determination whatsoever. A person would then be self-determined where she voluntarily lives a life according to her free choice; only where she does not choose freely, her self-determination would be in doubt.

The discussion about the concept of self-determination accordingly seems to oscillate between two philosophical poles: On one side, the ideal of perfectionism, which takes the development of potentials as a criterion for self-determination, and, on the other side, the ideal of voluntarism – as I call it – which only focuses on an individual's own selection of options. As it often happens, or so it seems to me, the most plausible approach lies somewhere between the two extremes.

In my analysis, I would hence like to illuminate the notion of self-determination a little more, not in pursuing any sort of conceptual analysis, but rather by discussing actual philosophical interpretations of this concept and weighing their arguments. First and foremost, I will defend a normative conception of self-determination. I believe the most plausible interpretation of self-determination necessarily encompasses an aspect of the right or good way of self-determination. In pursuing this argumentative goal my point of departure will be an equivocation that engenders two central aspects of the idea of self-determination: Self-determination can either mean to determine oneself in the world or it can mean to determine one's self. The possibility of the second sort of self-determination – which I will call self-formation – implies envisaging alternatives for one's own self that can be realised (cf. Bransen 2002). The mentioned alternatives of understanding self-determination, combined with the distinction between voluntarism and perfectionism, leads me to a four-fold categorisation of different theories of self-determination. In the following I will illustrate this classification with the help of philosophical theories devised by Harry Frankfurt, Thomas Hill Green and John Stuart Mill.

When I refer to "a self" in this paper, I merely mean to refer to the attributes, capabilities, value beliefs and characteristics of a person. I do not want to add a metaphysical claim about the ontology of selves (cf. Velleman 2006, 1). As far as I am concerned, selves are assemblages of aspects of an individual being. In addition, I want to presume that there is a self only where there is a relationship of a being to itself; where it can understand itself this or that way (cf. Taylor 1985). To this end it is important that such a being is conscious of itself and acquires knowledge about itself. The peculiar form of self-relation is an old theme of philosophy (cf. Taylor 1989), of course, but for my analysis it is only relevant in terms of representing a precondition of self-determination. My main aim is to clarify what it means to determine oneself and one's self.

## 3.2 Self-Actualisation and Self-Formation

As mentioned before, the concept of self-determination has two dimensions: The determination of decisions and actions by oneself and the determination of one's self. In most contexts self-determination is understood in the first sense, for instance when applied to the choices of patients in a medical context. They determine themselves in cases where they decide between therapeutic options and where this decision is actually implemented. Talk of self-determination as a determination of the self, i.e. self-determination in the second sense, is predominantly discussed in connection with the metaphysical problem of free will: In order for freedom of the will to be possible, some might claim, it is required that aspects of the self, for instance the character of a person, have been determined by the person herself and not arisen through some deterministic mechanism. For the sake of simplicity, I will from now on refer to self-determination as action under the aegis of oneself – self-determination in the first sense – as *self-actualisation* and to the determination of one's own self – self-determination in the second sense – as *self-formation*.

To illustrate the two ideas, one could claim that a student only self-determinedly or freely chose to study philosophy if the underlying desire itself was in turn determined or generated by that person herself. The willing student of philosophy might actualise herself by acting on her choice, but her respective will might not have been formed by herself. I believe many quarrels about people being or not being self-determined are due to cross-purposes regarding the two different ideas of self-determination.

Still, should we really accept this differentiation between two meanings of self-determination? Does is not lead to various philosophical dead ends, especially in terms of the metaphysical problem of free will? It seems to me that we can indeed make sense to the relevant distinction in a way that does not simply merge into the problem of free will. It appears to me that a focus on the debate regarding free will would put us on the wrong course. For it seems to pose the problem of self-determination in the following way: Self-determination is the actualisation of aspects of the self – desires, value judgments, personal characteristics, etc. – in the world; but how does the self, which determines itself here, arise? Was it determined by itself or "externally" determined? The problem with this point of view lies in the fact that existence of the self is postulated prior to its own actualisation.

This is a problematic point of view: according to it, first a self is developed, and this is then actualised through actions. The problem is that within such a framework we can ask the question whether one's self has been determined by oneself, which makes it obvious that a doubling of the self has arisen. There would have to be in turn someone, a self, who forms the self. The structure of self-determination as an actualisation in the world is transposed onto the self within this dubious framework; the self becomes the result of the forming actions of a – probably another – self. This view therefore produces a kind of homunculus that forms the person.

To be sure, these problems are by no means new, and especially in relation to the related philosophical problem of self-consciousness they have been well analysed (Tugendhat 1989). The questionable aspect stems from the translation of a subject-object structure into the idea of self-formation. In order to be able to "form" one-self – an object – there would have to be already to be a subject in place, which precedes the self to be formed. But here subject and object are of course identical, and herein lies the philosophical oddity.

The problem of the subject-object structure is relatively easy to solve. We should simply say that a person forms and expresses herself through her actions (Schechtman 2004). This framework circumvents the problematic implication of a split between a forming self, the "former", as it were, and that which is to be formed. There is accordingly no prior self, no homunculus. Insofar as we have different options there are also different possible self-formations.

In addition, this way of understanding self-formation allows "quality control"; in other words, assessments of right and wrong or good and bad self-formations. As we shall see, this is a central element of the philosophical discussion about self-determination: Human beings have an "evaluative self-relation" (Quante 2007, 29).

Yet understood in this way the difference between self-actualisation and self-formation indeed seems to collapse, for to actualise oneself now simply seems to mean to express one's self. To be sure, one could form oneself in various ways so long as one can act in varying ways, but there would seem to be no scope here for an incongruence between self-actualisation and self-formation. One would simply be what one expresses, or what one does.

This would be an unsatisfactory result in my opinion, since the relevant phenomenon of actualising oneself in a way that one is not, hence in a way that does not correspond to one's true self, is very real. One can be a person who does not express herself in the actions she commits. The person's actions in these cases are, as it is said, alienated or inauthentic (cf. Oshana 2010). Here the person is therefore not expressing herself qua self-determined actions; nonetheless she acts self-determinedly, in the sense that she actualises a self freely.

It seems implausible to me to completely abandon the concept of self-determination in those cases in which actions are alienated in order to maintain a conceptual identity between self-actualisation and self-formation. There are definitely forms of self-actualisation in which a person does not express *her self* and still acts self-determinedly. Indeed, the converse also seems possible: A person might express her own self in that she actualises herself; these are cases in which the person identifies with her actions. Here she determines herself (really), that is, here the congruence between self-formation and self-actualisation is present. This congruence seems to be the primary goal of self-determination: To express oneself through actions in the way that one sees oneself; which in turn means to act in harmony with oneself. Collapsing the idea of self-actualisation and self-formation seems to undermine our conceptual resources to describe and value these cases.

In my opinion we should therefore not level the difference between self-actualisation and self-formation, for we would remain on the level of factual description if we see congruence in each case. We could then do no more than indicate that a person is the one who actualises herself in free action; that is, we would have generated a purely descriptive concept of self-determination. The only relevant criterion of self-determination would be the exhibition of voluntary decisions and the corresponding options to act. Naturally I do not want to claim that this purely descriptive use of the expression "self-determination" would be pointless or useless. It does for instance function well in political philosophy, where the limits of legitimate influences on decisions are involved. Yet it seems to me that such a restricted view of the concept of self-determination neither fully captures the phenomena nor takes account of all ways of looking at related ethical problems.

The idea of self-formation implies the idea of alternative selves. We are not simply those who actualise themselves in decisions and free actions, but rather ones who have the possibility – however limited – to be this or that way. In brief, we can form ourselves within certain limits (cf. Glover 1988). We can also conceive of different alternatives of ourselves; we can for example imagine how it would be like to be more selfish or to live the life of an artist in the South Seas instead of with a family in the big city. We can also evaluate these alternatives. We can try to bring these hypothetical, alternative selves – let's call them self-ideals – into reality. In this way a potential incongruence arises between the actual self-actualisation and possible alternative forms of self-actualisation, that is to say, the actualisation of alternative selves. Here it is important to note that the difference between the actual self, which actualises itself in actions, and the self-ideal, which could be actualised in actions, does not lead to a problematic doubling of the self – criticised above – since here no synchronically present multiple selves are postulated.

With this differentiation we succeed in gaining a normative point of view in application to the concept of self-determination, for now we can ask how and towards what end we should determine ourselves. The goal in this pursuit is to reach a congruence between self-actualisation and self-ideal, that is, to express one's ideal self in self-determining actions.

Now we can return to the extreme positions of voluntarism and perfectionism that were mentioned at the beginning, so that four possibilities of conceiving self-determination arise:

1. Voluntarist Self-Actualisation: Self-determination means to actualise one's true self. This self is not created by the person herself, but is rather revealed through her actions. The point is to be what one is. The goal of self-determination is to be authentic.
2. Voluntarist Self-Formation: Self-determination means to actualise one's chosen self. The point is to make oneself that which one has chosen oneself to be. The goal of self-determination is to actualise one's own self-conception.
3. Perfectionist Self-Actualisation: Self-determination means to become one's best possible self, to actualise one's potentials. The point is to become the most developed variation of oneself that one can be.
4. Perfectionist Self-Formation: Self-determination means to actualise the best possible self. The point is to become the most developed variation of a self that is possible.

It barely needs emphasising that this categorisation has its own problems. It will nevertheless serve to bring order into the upcoming examples of philosophical theories and hopefully to help making progress in the discussion on self-determination. I refer to the philosophical theories I discuss as theories of self-determination, even if the concept of self-determination is not central to all the respective theories. As shall be seen, I refer to Harry Frankfurt's approach as a version of voluntarist self-actualisation. The problem of his reflections seems to me primarily to lie in that he leaves no room for a self-ideal that departs from the mere being-identical-with-oneself. Thomas Hill Green, who represents the perfectionist self-formation version, has, as it were, a little too much of this idea of the ideal self. He lays out an ideal self that is not one's own self, but is rather attained from the outside by reference to the idea of reason. In John Stuart Mill we find an ideal of one's self that is thoroughly one's own self; a self which does not lie outside of the self-relation of the person, hence is not self-formed, yet can be improved. Mill therefore represents the perfectionist self-actualisation version. This approach seems to me most plausible and I will defend it up to a certain point. The voluntarist self-formation version, which can perhaps be connected most closely to Jean-Paul Sartre, will not be discussed here. To me this approach is a non-starter, because it either reproduces the homunculus-problem or, in any plausible variation, in which a person actualises herself as the self she has formed, collapses into either of the two self-actualisation variants.

## 3.3 Self-Identification: Harry Frankfurt's Theory of Voluntarist Self-Actualisation

According to Frankfurt, a specific capacity of persons is to turn desires into objects of our volitions (Frankfurt 1971). We can accordingly take a stance with respect to ourselves in that we may desire to be effectively motivated through specific desires. Desires in this model are hierarchically structured; we can evaluate desires of the first order and thereby generate desires of a second order – desires with respect to desires. This is in no way a strange philosophical idea, but is rather in line with everyday experience, for instance when we, starting from a desire to eat chocolate, distance ourselves and desire instead that the particular action may not be initiated.

In Frankfurt's account, a person acts from her own will when the effectively motivating desires are the ones that she desires to be motivated by; hence if a person's so-called second-order volitions are actualized. For our purposes we might want to say that second-order desires represent an element of the self-ideal of a person. This self-ideal does not actualize itself in each case of action. For numerous reasons an incongruence can arise between the way in which one actually determines oneself and the way in which one desires to determine oneself. If a person however identifies herself with the desire that has a motivating effect on actions – that is, the "will" in Frankfurt's terminology – then she acts on account of her *own* will. This, according to Frankfurt, means to enjoy free will (Frankfurt 1971, 17).

But on which basis does one identify with certain desires? Structurally, within Frankfurt's model, it is second-order volitions that serve this function of identification, but from where do these stem? Are they self-chosen and thereby, potentially anyway, brought under the hierarchical model? This would require a possibly infinite regress in the structure of desires; that is, even higher-order volitions than the second-order ones. Frankfurt's answer is that the continuation of the volitional hierarchy ends where one wholeheartedly identifies with a desire (Frankfurt 1987). Accordingly, action-controlling desires – representing the will – are not always themselves objects of wilful identification. In other words, in the case of decisive identification there is no considered choice between different first-order desires, rather, when acting wholeheartedly, the will is simply based on the personal characteristics one happens to have.

For a person, it can lie at the heart to act one way and not another; and then it appears unthinkable to her to have another will. Although this almost sounds like a description of compulsive behaviour, according to Frankfurt a person is nevertheless not acting unfreely in this case. On the contrary, she then acts on her *own* free will – on what she cares about – because she identifies herself wholeheartedly with the motivating desire. Such an identification does not lead her to any further weighing or reasoning – a kind of undecidedness – but rather to a satisfaction with a given configuration of the will (cf. Seel 2002, 291f.)

When developing his theory, Frankfurt later went even further and introduced the notion of volitional necessities (Frankfurt 1982). In a supposedly paradoxical way, volitional necessities become the epitome of freedom, because through them we act wholeheartedly on the basis of our own will. The necessitating character of these special volitions in turn inhibits the ascent into higher spheres of volition – it ends all questioning and balancing about motivating desires' adequacy or justification. Since no assessment of desires is possible in these circumstances – after all a person is then driven by a form of compulsion – there is no scope for an infinite progress of hierarchies of volition.

Frankfurt even describes the phenomenon of love within this model: Its will-defining necessities signify culmination points within the structure of caring. "Loving is a mode of caring. Among the things that we care about there are some that we cannot help caring about; and among the things that we cannot help caring about are those that we love" (Frankfurt 1999, 165).

However, Frankfurt has created a new problem with his analysis, one that has garnered much criticism: Volitional necessities cannot really be objects of a person's own evaluation, because they are not really available to the person; they have no control over volitional necessities. Yet this means that the very possibility of subjective critical engagement with any of one's wholehearted desires has apparently been ignored by Frankfurt. Such a model seems to leave out something rather important: the critique of oneself as regards one's basic commitments. Frankfurt insists on a model of self-determination that builds on reflexivity – desires regarding desires – without reflection – a critical stance towards oneself (cf. Christman 1991b; Herrmann 2000, 159).

Accordingly, in Frankfurt's model, whether a person acts in unity with her own will is ultimately determined merely by a specific volitional relation, namely a strong identification between volitions. Self-determination is hence independent of what would be intelligent, rational or morally imperative – independent of any subject-external normative standard. Frankfurt indeed insists that it is the very unavailable subjective will that forms reasons for actions, and not the other way around – that is, reasons forming the will. In an alternative model, where a person would weigh and assess reasons for or against a specific action, she would require, according to Frankfurt, prior evaluative criteria. Yet, these criteria themselves can only be based on the person's own wholehearted commitments.

> This means that the most basic and essential question for a person to raise concerning the conduct of his life cannot be the *normative* question of how he *should* live. That question can sensibly be asked only on the basis of a prior answer to the *factual* question of what he actually *does* care about (Frankfurt 2004, 26; emphasis in original).

For Frankfurt, the concern about something is the source of reasons. We cannot justify what we care about, only uncover it, for we are "beings, who do not create themselves" (Frankfurt 2004, 20). To be sure, Frankfurt does in no way want to exclude that the worthiness of an object can causally produce or influence caring or love. But in order to really be able to love something or someone, this behaviouristic basis is not sufficient to produce worthy volitions, since a person must individually be able to actualise – to live, as it were – a particular object of love or concern. "It is not necessarily as a *result* of recognizing their value and of being captivated by it that we love things. Rather, what we love necessarily *acquires* value for us *because* we love it" (Frankfurt 2004, 38f.; emphasis in original). The desirable or valuable object has to possess an attractive power for the lover. Therefore, an unavoidably personal element is found in love. We show ourselves in what we love.

It seems to me that there are very significant insights regarding the concept of self-determination within Frankfurt's model of the will structure, even in the supposedly overstretched idea of volitional necessity. The capacity for self-determination touches upon our capacity to enter a position towards ourselves. We act self-determinedly if we can actualise the conception of our self in the world with which we identify ourselves. Our freedom appears exactly at that point, when we are determined in a special way from the bottom of our hearts, or through aspects about which we are most concerned. The point of self-determination is not to actualise a supposedly free, self-produced will, but rather our *own* will.

Yet Frankfurt's strict rejection of any reflection about the question as to how one should live or rather what kind of person one should be, independently of the question of what one is content with, indeed seems excessive. He seems to be driven by a concern, which is internal to his theory, to avoid the potential infinite regress of his hierarchical model of volition. Yet it is a common experience of human beings that we are not only able to take a stance towards our motivating desires, but also in relation to deep-rooted aspects of ourselves. When we determine ourselves, then we are always – however indirectly – concerned with the right ways, or at least with alternative ways, of self-determination.

Few people would generally be satisfied with a simple "I am what I am" – even if that might be enough for their daily lives. Our self, that is, our attributes, evaluative beliefs, motivations, etc., is not clearly predefined. We can always think of new alternatives to it. Even if Frankfurt rightly emphasises that we should be concerned with realising ourselves in the form in which we are contented with ourselves, this does not mean that we could not very well have reasons nonetheless to imagine ourselves differently and perhaps even to hold these images as being better for us. We can foster desires for alternatives to what kind of person we are. Frankfurt's philosophical concern regarding the hierarchical structure of his model seems to be unfounded: The decision in what way or to what end we should actualise ourselves does not require a third order of volition, although it does require some kind of consideration.

To be sure, Frankfurt rightly questions the idea of a wilful formation of one's own self. Perhaps we merely delude ourselves when we assume that we would have the possibility to form ourselves in our deep-rooted aspects. To illuminate this problem further, I will elaborate on the idea of the formation of one's own self in the following section.

## 3.4 Self-Realisation: Thomas Hill Green's Ideal of Perfectionist Self-Formation

Before discussing Green, it helps to introduce a famous critic of his account, who has unfortunately dented Green's philosophical reputation for some time. Isaiah Berlin, in his famous Oxford inaugural lecture *Two Concepts of Liberty*, objects to an ideal concept of liberty, and he ascribes this idea mainly to Green. Even if in this work Berlin does not explicitly use the concept of self-determination, it is clear that his discussion is pertinent to the interpretation I have pursued so far (Berlin 2002, 53). For Berlin the problematic idea of positive freedom results from asking the already mentioned question whether a person is indeed herself that person who forms herself. In Berlin's own words: whether one is master over one's own self (Berlin 2002, 178).

In this way Berlin also seems to reject any normatively conceived conception of the correct or best way of self-determination or of the exercise of freedom, because such a normative account seems to come with an ideal of rational or moral self-determination. For instance, he endorses Bentham's rhetorical question: "The liberty of doing evil, is it not liberty?" (Berlin 2002, 194). To be sure, I do not believe that Berlin therefore has to accept every possible form of actual self-determination as unproblematic and as the right form for the particular person; this does not seem for instance to be the case if a person is ignorant about what is in reality contributing to her own good.

But Berlin does not seem to allow for there to be incongruence between the self that is actually expressed in actions and another form of self-actualisation that could result from an alternative account of one's self. Berlin is quite careful not to commit to postulate alternative selves, even where he wants to allow criticism of some exercises of freedom (Berlin 2002, 41, 177). In my terminology, it might be said that when he explains the possibility of criticising self-actualisation, he avoids any possibility of self-formation. Yet in this regard he seems to be going too far, for he thereby dismisses the possibility of differentiating between the actual self-actualisation in particular actions and a possible alternative self-actualisation in line with a self-ideal.

This is a problem for Berlin, because not every conception of ideal self-actualisation seems to necessarily take on the problematic form that Berlin dismisses, namely to be determined to a degree by a conception of the "'real' self, of which the poor empirical self in space and time may know nothing or little" (Berlin 2002, 180). To this extent the differentiation between various ways of self-actualisation and their evaluations would not be problematic as such, even according to Berlin, but rather the specific form of this differentiation, which is assumed in theories that take as a basis a subject-external ideal, for instance on grounds of an account of specific human purposes. Berlin therefore seems to accept forms of "quality control" of self-determination, but he dismisses normative considerations of how – or in which way – we should determine ourselves. Yet exactly here lies the flaw of Berlin's argument, for it means to dismiss the underlying practical question of how one is to live. To omit this very aspect seems inadequate when it comes to a theory of self-determination (cf. Gerhardt 1999).

British philosopher Thomas Hill Green, who was strongly influenced by Hegel, is one of the best-known proponents of a conception of positive freedom. As mentioned, he is also one of the antagonists of Berlin's defence of negative freedom, which merely requires the absence of coercion. Green, in contrast to Berlin, is of the belief that freedom consists in determining oneself in a particular way.

It needs to be stressed that Green does not commit the previously discussed error of assuming a kind of homunculus in order to differentiate between actual and right ways of determining oneself. His point is accordingly not to iteratively ask whether the will that actualises itself in actions could itself count as free. Locke had already brushed off this question as meaningless in his *Essay Concerning Human*

*Understanding*, and Green shares this view. The will as such is *by definition* free, because human beings express themselves in executions of their will; indeed, Green describes the figure of speech "free will" as a pleonasm (Green 1879, 308). In this respect Berlin's critique of Green has to be challenged, since it depends on the assumption that when using the concept of positive freedom one need to presume that there is an agency – the "dominant self"– that rules over the will, or the "empirical self" (Berlin 2002, 179f.). Green however maintains: "The will is simply the man" (Green 1883, 158). Accordingly, Green postulates no synchronic reduplication of the self, even when he talks about being "master of himself" (Green 1879, 322). To be the master of oneself does not mean to be a self that has a master, who is identical to oneself.

> There is no such thing as a will which a man is not conscious of as belonging to himself, no such thing as an act of will which he is not conscious of as issuing from himself. To ask whether he has power over it, or whether some other power than he determines it, is like asking whether he is other than himself. Thus the question whether a man, having power to act according to his will, or being free to act, has also power over his will, or is free to will, has just the same impropriety that Locke points out in the question whether the will is free (Green 1879, 317f.).

Green distinguishes between freedom in the "juristic" or civil sense – the negative freedom of Berlin's – and a freedom that represents a certain form of self-formation (Green 1879, 315), whereby this form allows different interpretations: The formation of oneself according to nature, as the Stoics assumed; according to God's will like in Paul; in the sense of a universal lawgiver as in Kant; or pursuant of the interests of a well-regulated state like in Hegel. For Green himself, the best result of self-determination consists in realising a specific version of an ideal self. To discuss this ideal, he indeed uses the notion of positive freedom, but for him this positive freedom is based on negative freedom. In this regard positive freedom therefore does not stand in opposition to Berlin's approach.

> [T]o the grown man, bred to civil liberty in a society which has learnt to make nature its instrument, there is no self-enjoyment in the mere consciousness of freedom as exemption from external control, no sense of an object in which he can satisfy himself having been obtained. […] 'freedom' is the natural term by which the man describes such an object to himself, – describes to himself the state in which he shall have realised his ideal of himself […] (Green 1879, 323f.).

The will therefore has to lead to a specific goal in order for a person (in this positive sense) to be able to be free: The improvement, and eventually the perfection, of herself. There is nothing philosophically strange at all in this idea. Berlin was of course concerned about the possible political consequences of such a conception, which could come close to forcing people to achieve the relevant perfection. But nothing in Green's account as such seems to imply these potentially coercive measures (cf. Geuss 1995). His approach is indeed in harmony with my previous observations, for Green's point is to hold firm that the idea of self-determination always includes possibilities or potentials and that a driving force of human beings consists in realising these potentials: "[Man] has the impulse to make himself what he has the possibility of becoming but actually is not […]" (Green 1883, 182).

The problems that Berlin pointed out begin where such an ideal is forced onto persons and does not even represent a person's own ideal self. To be sure, at least on the face of it, for Green the idea consists in purely formal aspects, so does not seem to impose a particular interpretation of the ideal self. To the extent that one can control oneself through the operation of one's practical reason, the perfection of oneself consists in the best possible operation of the capabilities connected with reason (cf. Simhony 1993).

The label Green introduces for this idea, especially in the posthumously published *Prolegomena to Ethics*, is "self-realisation" (cf. Brink 2003, 41). Yet the realisation of the self in Green's approach does not appear to be a realisation of one's *own* self after all. It rather consists in the realisation of the best possible self that is determined on the basis of criteria that are not our own, but stem from a theory of the rational nature of human beings. In this respect, Berlin's worries seem well-founded. "Once I take this view, I am in a position to ignore the actual wishes of men or societies, to bully, oppress, torture them in the name, and on behalf, of their 'real' selves, in the secure knowledge that whatever is the true goal of man" (Berlin 2002, 180).

In addition, the notion of self-realisation has connotations that cast doubt on the very idea of actualising one's own potentials. 'Self-realisation' seems to be referring to the realisation of that which is already present in the self. To which extent are ideal alternatives of our selves actually available to us? To which extent is it in our power to form ourselves? If we cannot form ourselves according to an ideal of the self, then Green's theory is potentially vacuous. A philosophical theory that allows insights regarding the restricted scope for self-formation is that of John Stuart Mill.

## 3.5 Self-Development: John Stuart Mill's Conception of Perfectionist Self-Actualisation

It may be surprising to suggest that Mill puts in doubt the possibility of human beings to form themselves, since he is generally supposed to be a proponent of a fairly radical liberalism that wants to see individual freedom as broadly protected as possible. Why protect something that cannot really be achieved? Yet liberalism involves first and foremost a perspective on the societal and political conditions of self-determination in the sense of self-actualisation. One can reasonably want to protect self-determination without believing in the possibility of the independent formation of alternative selves. Political liberalism as such is non-committal about the feasibility of self-formation. If the idea were rejected, the point of political provisions to protect self-determination would then be to model them in a way that an already laid out or latent self can develop. Mill seems to suggest exactly this approach when he compares self-development with the growing of a tree: "Human nature is not a machine to be built after a model, and set to do exactly the work prescribed for it, but a tree, which requires to grow and develop itself on all sides, according to the tendency of the inward forces which make it a living thing." (Mill 1859, 263). The inward forces here might very well be interpreted as the specific characteristics of a pre-conceived individual self.

In contrast to Green, Mill does not speak of self-realisation, but rather of self-development, although it – so it seems – could terminologically have come the other way around, since Green's account involves perfection and Mill refers to the realisation of inner forces. Obviously this choice of terms has, at least in Green's case, philosophical-historical reasons and goes back to his reference to Hegel. Be that as it may, in the quoted passage Mill indeed sounds as if he allows self-formation only little scope. A tree just cannot decide in which direction it wants to grow, although its growth is influenced through its environment and not completely determined by inherent forces. Self-determination, within this picture, would consequently be merely the actualisation of an already existing, latent self. To be sure, a person could still act inauthentically, for instance when she does something against her own nature only because the majority of people do it. She then acted, according to Mill, not as an individual, but rather as a member of a herd. Individuality requires in his opinion having one's own idea of how one should live. The point of self-development is therefore to actualise *one's own* self. Yet this very self seems again to be something to be discovered, not created or formed.

Understood this way, Mill's theory seems unpromising because the development of one's own potentials alone seems deficient as an ideal of self-determination. Consider Sisyphus: His potential – though admittedly forced upon him by the gods – consisted in again and again hauling a stone up a hill. Would the development of this potential already be a worthwhile way to self-determination? Now, Sisyphus could develop this single ability, which still remains for him to actualise. Joel Feinberg speculates accordingly: "[T]he gods might have designed for him a peculiar talent for rockpushing much like others' talents for pianoplaying, tennis, or chess. The new Sisyphus starts all over as a perpetual youth, and from the start he is a veritable prodigy at rockpushing. He comes to enjoy exercising his skills, and makes evernew challenges for himself. He pushes the rock righthanded, then lefthanded, then nohanded, then blindfolded, then does two at a time, then juggles three in the air all the way to the summit, eager to return for another so that he can break his record" (Feinberg 1980, 320). Most people would likely regard the life of a perfect stone-hauler as an absurd form of self-realisation, even if – contrary to the actual example – Sisyphus had himself chosen the occupation of a stone-hauler. This sentiment is likely based in the belief that the practice of certain capabilities cannot represent a reasonable self-ideal, and that their actualisation therefore also facilitates no proper form of self-determination.

So far, we have interpreted Mill's idea of self-development as restricted to pre-conceived individual characteristics. Yet Mill's conception of discovering one's own self in order to live self-determinedly allows two possible interpretations: On the one hand the point of self-determination could be to discover in each case one's own nature, that is, the essence of each individual, and to actualise this in the world. Here the concept of authenticity would be appropriate, since it is applied to describe the relation of an individual to itself. On the other hand, it would be conceivable that

Mill postulates a general nature of human beings, which in turn would be there to be discovered in self-actualisation. Here we would not be speaking of authenticity, but perhaps of self-emergence – since it is here that a person altogether comes to a specifically human way of life.

Mill is renowned for his deliberations on individual diversity and originality, up to a defence of human eccentricity. In this regard the first interpretation appears pertinent, whereupon self-determination is the actualisation of a unique self; a "quiddity" (Gray 1991, 193). Accordingly Mill emphasizes the value of pluralism of "experiments in living" (Mill 1859, 281). In this interpretation there appears to be no normative standard of a right self-determination: The point simply is to actualise oneself as one is. The authentic Sisyphus or the authentic Dude, to use the former example, would from this point of view be self-determined human beings.

If, however, we refer to other works, especially Mill's account of hedonism in *Utilitarianism*, it is clear, at least to my mind, that also the second interpretation, i.e. the assumption of specific human aspects of self-development, was not foreign to Mill. For there he claimed that a genuinely human life would be preferable to a "pig-like" life (Mill 1861, 210ff.). In these passages Mill sounds Aristotelian and hence perfectionist – there are according to him bad kinds of self-actualisation after all, because they violate the ideal form of a human life. "Few human creatures would consent to be changed into any of the lower animals, for a promise of the fullest allowance of a beast's pleasures; no intelligent human being would consent to be a fool, no instructed person would be an ignoramus, no person of feeling and conscience would be selfish and base, even though they should be persuaded that the fool, the dunce, or the rascal is better satisfied with his lot than they are with theirs" (Mill 1861, 211).

The two interpretations of Mill's account of self-determination do not in any way have to contradict each other: One can indeed postulate a general human form of self-development and simultaneously be of the opinion that every person qua self-determining being develops her own individual version of this general human nature, i.e. forms herself into an individual person. The only case where these two accounts conflicted would be where an individual way of life would to some extent be unhuman. For Mill, this extreme case seems to imply that it does not involve genuine self-determination. Whether this again is a philosophically dubious proposition depends first and foremost on how narrow the perfectionist framework, which Mill builds, actually is. Although I cannot elaborate on this question here, it seems clear to me that the point for Mill is to reveal forms of merely alleged self-determination that deny the underlying human capabilities. His point was not to establish specific ways of life as the only appropriate ones for humans; that would also contradict his belief in the "unlikeness of one person to another" (Mill 1859, 273) in connection with his notion that to develop oneself is only possible where one lives one's own life.

Surely it is empirically possible, according to Mill, that one does not actualise underlying human capabilities, or does not want to actualise them, and therefore lives against human nature, somewhat like a pig. Yet it would just not be desirable – Mill can make that claim, for he proposes a normative conception of self-determination. At the same time this framework does not involve more than the claim that self-determination shall lead to a life that achieves the predicate "human". Within this frame there remains a variety of good ways of individual self-development. In summary, the scope for self-formation is limited by an account of the proper form of human nature, yet the scope is still wide and allows for individuality.

There is still the question whether Mill allows for self-formation. It seems that certain aspects of human nature by and large elude human control in his account. To be sure, he merely seems to imply that we cannot determine the contours of the appropriate frame of self-determination, properly understood, for this is given to us as human nature. To properly determine oneself it is necessary to stay within this frame. At the same time, we individually actualise ourselves within these contours because we understand it as a task or responsibility, not because we are forced, that is, determined by the laws of nature. It is necessary to choose the right goals, namely those that do not defraud a human life. This means to form oneself according to one's own ideal within self-endorsed limits.

This conception still allows the possibility to form oneself as a unique individual. Individuality in this understanding does not solely consist in affirming through choice exactly those characteristics which our individual nature specifies for us. In his work *A System of Logic*, of which the sixth book is dedicated to the "logic of the moral sciences", Mill takes to task the fatalistic argument whereby the character of a person "is formed *for* him, and not *by* him" (Mill 1843, 840, emphasis in original; cf. Evans 2007, 61ff.) and that it would therefore be useless to desire that it was cultivated in a different way. To this Mill replies: "But this is a grand error. He has, to a certain extent, a power to alter his character. Its being, in the ultimate resort, formed for him, is not inconsistent with its being, in part, formed *by* him as one of the intermediate agents. His character is formed by his circumstances (including among these his particular organization); but his own desire to mould it in a particular way, is one of those circumstances, and by no means one of the least influential" (Mill 1843, 840, emphasis in original).

So according to Mill, the desire to cultivate and educate one's self is essential for self-formation. But how does this desire in turn come about? Is it accessible to us? Mill grapples with this last fatalistic objection: "But to think that we have no power of altering our character, and to think that we shall not use our power unless we desire to use it, are very different things, and have a very different effect on the mind. A person who does not wish to alter his character, cannot be the person who is supposed to feel discouraged or paralysed by thinking himself unable to do it. The depressing effect of the fatalist doctrine can only be felt where there *is* a wish to do what that doctrine represents as impossible" (Mill 1843, 841, emphasis in original).

It therefore doesn't matter whether the desire to form oneself was itself again determined; it matters whether it is present. We have to conceive of ourselves as self-forming beings; only then can we be satisfied or unsatisfied with ourselves. The fatalist cannot at all account for the common distinction between those who live under the aegis of necessity and those who live under the aegis of freedom. We have already seen before that self-determination does not mean to have a self that is brought forward through one's own choice. Self-determination means, also according to Mill, to actualise oneself in the world in the way one would like to. Now to still ask the question whether having chosen freely the way one would like to be means asking too much.

However, an important problem indeed, which fatalists could draw attention to and which is connected to the idea of authenticity, seems to be the following: Up until now we have expressed the idea of self-determination such that a person forms herself in that she expresses herself in actions, value beliefs etc. In addition, there was the idea of a self-ideal, which can bring us to conceive of other actions, value beliefs etc. to form ourselves in other ways. Yet, on this basis, how shall we explain the phenomenon that it can happen that a person never, or at least extremely rarely, expresses herself in actions in a way that corresponds to her self-ideal? In other words, on what basis can someone claim to be rather someone else, an ideal version of herself, if she never expresses this ideal version of herself in reality?

An example shall illuminate this consideration: Assume that a person who maintains herself to be orderly and meticulous carries out activities that are consistently sloppy. Can this person reasonably claim that she is actually completely different – namely orderly and meticulous – but for whatever reasons consistently acts inauthentically; that is that she is permanently "out of character"? In order to be able to really act inauthentically, so it seems, there has to be at least evidence of another possible self in a person. Whether this alternative self exists seems in turn not to be entirely a matter of the person, but also to a substantial degree depend on the assessment of others. If, for example, others never experience a person as polite, then she is not polite. Surely she can strive to become more polite, but to claim that she is not really herself when she is impolite seems in these circumstances inconceivable.

The idea of authenticity depends on the possible incongruence between the factual self-actualisation and another way to determine oneself, which supposedly better actualises the self. A distinction between actual and possible self-actualisation therefore makes philosophical sense. Where single actions contradict observably consistent characteristics of a person, judgements of inauthenticity indeed seem to be justified. Yet self-ideals cannot be determined fully detached from how a person really actualises herself. I do not mean to imply, of course, that people can never change themselves – only they have to change themselves first before they can reasonably claim that they do not show their true selves when they trespass against their own ideals. In brief: A Saul might change himself into a Paul. But Paul cannot claim that he did not actualise himself as Saul.

In summary, Mill's account helps us to see that the idea of self-formation needs to be closely linked to the idea of self-actualisation. We can form ourselves, but we always need to evidence it in expressions of our self. At the same time, Mill's account stands for the perfectionist idea of improvement of character. For him, there is a shape of a human life-form, which we need to endorse if we want to really be self-determined. Within these contours, we can become an individual; our very own person.

## 3.6 Conclusion

Let us summarise what has resulted in the course of this analysis. Self-determination does not merely mean to actualise a self, but also to scrutinise whether someone actualises oneself in the way that he or she wants to be or should be. This *should* seems to me to always be understood in a hypothetical sense, not categorical, since it is bound to the perspective of the person herself, insofar as the point is realising an *own* self (cf. Christman 1991a). An ideal self that only comes from the outside, with which one then does not identify, cannot fulfil this criterion. Hence self-determination can be understood as a normative concept. Human beings have aspirations that allow them to describe alternatives to themselves and to strive towards these alternatives (cf. Gewirth 1998). In this regard incongruences can appear between the self that one expresses in decisions and actions and the self that one wants to be.

Additionally the possibility arises – which Harry Frankfurt appears to ignore – that we are the ones who we want to be – or to be more precise: that we are content with ourselves – and yet at the same time foster alternative self-ideals, because we see reasons to be different. There is no contradiction involved between acting wholeheartedly and still striving to be different: In the same way that we can be content with different lives, we have the possibility to foster different self-ideals in ourselves, towards each of which we can attempt to strive. We do not need a sophisticated theory for how to choose or how we should choose between these alternative selves. It is enough to acknowledge that we can actualise ourselves in different ways and that we can take a stance towards the specific way and the goal of our self-actualisation. We identify ourselves with our decisions and actions not merely on the grounds of a preconceived idea of who we are, but rather evaluate this self on the grounds of simultaneously available alternative ideas of who we could be. There appears to be little that can be said regarding to which extent these alternative selves are available to us. On the one hand we know that human beings can change drastically, and on the other hand a self-ideal to be actualised should still be one's own self.

It also does not seem to me to be once and for all clear to which extent we should better ourselves in order to determine ourselves in the right way, or in order to become our best selves. In a negative fashion one could agree with Mill that at least the lower threshold set by general norms of self-development – those of human nature – restricts the proper scope of self-determination. But the assumption that one must also actualise individual potentials as best as possible seems to me to go too far.

I have called Mill's version of self-determination perfectionist self-actualisation. Labelled in this way, it presents an ideal-type position within a categorisation that mainly serves to organise the field of philosophical theories. When discussing Mill's theory more closely, it becomes clear that it does not allow for any simple categorisation after all. It is perfectionist only in a limited sense, as it leaves a large degree of leeway to subjective ideas as to how it is best to live. Even if it is first and foremost a theory of self-actualisation, its approach also remains obligated to the idea of self-formation. When we put together the best elements of the discussed theories, it appears to me that the proper way of self-determination consists in developing one's own human potentials as far as one oneself would like, in addition to realising these potentials in decisions and actions.

**Acknowledgements** I would like to thank Fabian Wendt, Andrea Esser and participants at the "Thick (Concepts of) Autonomy" conference in Münster (2012) and at the University of Arizona (2014) for helpful comments. This paper is a revised version of an article published in German in *Deutsche Zeitschrift für Philosophie* in 2011.

## References

Berlin, Isaiah. 2002. Two Concepts of Liberty. In *Liberty: Incorporating Four Essays on Liberty*, ed. Henry Hardy, 166–217. Oxford: Oxford University Press.
Bransen. Jan. 2002. Making and Finding Ourselves. In *Personal and Moral Identity*, ed. Albert W. Musschenga et al., 77–96. Dordrecht: Springer.
Brink, David O. 2003. *Perfectionism and the Common Good: Themes in the Philosophy of T. H. Green*. Oxford: Oxford University Press.
Christman, John. 1991a. Liberalism and Individual Positive Freedom. *Ethics* 101 (2): 343–359.
———. 1991b. Autonomy and Personal History. *Canadian Journal of Philosophy* 21 (1): 1–24.
Evans, Mark. 2007. *Self-Realization: Politics and the Good Life in Modern Times*. New York: Nova Science Publishers Inc.
Feinberg, Joel. 1980. Absurd Self-Fulfillment. In *Freedom and Fulfillment: Philosophical Essays*, 297–330. Princeton University Press 1992: Princeton.
Frankfurt, Harry. 1971. Freedom of the Will and the Concept of a Person. *Journal of Philosophy* 68 (1): 5–20.
———. 1982. The Importance of What We Care About. In *The Importance of What We Care About*, 80–94. Cambridge: Cambridge University Press 1988.
———. 1987. Identification and wholeheartedness. In *The importance of what we care about*, 159–176. Cambridge: Cambridge University Press 1988.
———. 1999. On Caring. In *Necessity, Volition, and Love*, 155–180. Cambridge: Cambridge University Press.
———. 2004. *The Reasons of Love*. Princeton: Princeton University Press.
Gerhardt, Volker. 1999. *Selbstbestimmung: Das Prinzip der Individualität* [Self-Determination: The Principle of Individuality]. Stuttgart: Reclam.
Geuss, Raymond. 1995. Freedom as an Ideal. *Proceedings of the Aristotelian Society*, Supplementary Volume 69: 87–100.
Gewirth, Alan. 1998. *Self-Fulfillment*. Princeton.
Glover, Jonathan. 1988. *I: The Philosophy and Psychology of Personal Identity*. London: Penguin.
Gray, John. 1991. Mill's Conception of Happiness and the Theory of Individuality. In *J.S. Mill: On Liberty in Focus*, ed. J. Gray and G.W. Smith, 190–211. London: Routledge.
Green, Thomas Hill. 1879. On the Different Senses of 'Freedom' as Applied to Will and to the Moral Progress of Man. In *The Works of Thomas Hill Green*, ed. P. Nicholson, vol. II, 308–333. London: Thoemmes Continuum 1997.
———. 1883. Prologomena to Ethics. In *The Works of Thomas Hill Green*, ed. P. Nicholson, vol. IV, 1–427. London: Thoemmes Continuum 1997.
Herrmann, Martina. 2000. Freier Wille ohne Wunschkritik – Autonomie als Zustimmung zum eigenen Wünschen [Free Will without Critiquing Desires – Autonomy as Affirmation of

Own Desires]. In *Autonomes Handeln: Beiträge zur Philosophie von Harry G. Frankfurt*, ed. M. Betzler and B. Guckes, 153–166. Berlin: Akademie.
Mill, John Stuart. 1843. A System of Logic. Ratiocinative and Inductive Part II. In *Collected Works*, ed. J.M. Robson, vol. VIII. Toronto: Toronto University Press 1969.
———. 1859. On Liberty. In *Collected Works*, ed. J.M. Robson, vol. XVIII, 213–310. Toronto: Toronto University Press 1977.
———. 1861. Utilitarianism. In *Collected Works*, ed. J.M. Robson, vol. X, 203–259. Toronto: Toronto University Press 1969.
Oshana, Marina. 2010. *The Importance of How We See Ourselves: SelfIdentity and Responsible Agency*. Lanham: Lexington Books.
Quante, Michael. 2007. *Person*. Berlin/New York: de Gruyter.
Rawls, John. 1999. *A Theory of Justice*. Revised ed. Cambridge, MA: Harvard University Press.
Schechtman, Marya. 2004. SelfExpression and SelfControl. *Ratio* 17 (4): 409–427.
Seel, Martin. 2002. Sich bestimmen lassen: Ein revidierter Begriff der Selbstbestimmung [To Let Oneself be Determined: A Revised Concept of Self-Determination]. In *Sich bestimmen lassen: Studien zur theoretischen und praktischen Philosophie*, 279–298. Frankfurt/M: Suhrkamp.
Simhony, Avital. 1993. Beyond Negative and Positive Freedom: T.H. Green's View of Freedom. *Political Theory* 21 (1): 28–54.
Taylor, Charles. 1985. SelfInterpreting Animals. In *Human Agency and Language*, Philosophical Papers I, 45–76. Cambridge: Cambridge University Press.
———. 1989. *Sources of the Self: The Making of the Modern Identity*. Cambridge: Cambridge University Press.
Tugendhat, Ernst. 1989. *Self-consciousness and Self-Determination*. Cambridge, MA: MIT Press.
Velleman, David. 2006. *Self to Self: Selected Essays*. Cambridge: Cambridge University Press.

# Chapter 4
# Self-Confidence, Self-Assertiveness, and Self-Esteem: The Triple S Condition of Personal Autonomy

**Johann S. Ach and Arnd Pollmann**

**Abstract** In this paper we seek to clarify the question of what exactly is meant by an "autonomous" decision or act by focusing on the most fundamental personal condition for deciding or acting autonomously. This basic personal requirement has often been overlooked in recent debates; where it has been seen, it is characterized in ways that are too demanding. What is meant here is an individual form of self-relation that seems to be constitutive for leading a life as a human and is likely to be acquired (or not) very early in life. This significant personal self-relation has three essential aspects: a primal sense of "self-confidence", a basic form of "self-assertiveness", and a fundamental form of "self-esteem". We will call this the "triple S condition" for autonomy. Our main thesis is that any decision or action which is not based on this triple S condition cannot be called "autonomous".

In bioethical discussions the normative principle of respect for the autonomy of patients plays a key role. However, even if the great normative significance of autonomy of the patient can now be considered as widely accepted, there is still controversy around a number of issues concerning the principle of autonomy. Especially open to dispute is the question of what exactly is meant by an autonomous decision or action, i.e. what makes an action *autonomous*. What are the descriptive criteria for autonomous actions?

In the following contribution we concentrate on one especially basic condition for autonomous decisions or actions that is often overlooked in discussion or, when seen, often characterized in a way that is too demanding. What is meant is a basic form of practical *self-relation* that has three essential aspects: a primal sense of "self-confidence", a basic form of active "self-assertiveness", and a just as fundamental form of "self-esteem". We will call this "the triple S condition" for

J. S. Ach (✉)
Center for Bioethics, Münster University, Münster, Germany
e-mail: ach@uni-muenster.de

A. Pollmann
Alice Salomon Hochschule Berlin, Berlin, Germany
e-mail: pollmann@ash-berlin.eu



J. F. Childress, M. Quante (eds.), *Thick (Concepts of) Autonomy*, Philosophical Studies Series 146, https://doi.org/10.1007/978-3-030-80991-1_4

autonomy, and our main thesis will be that any decision or action not based on this triple S condition cannot be called "autonomous".

## 4.1 The Standard Model for Autonomous Action

What must be the case in order to say that any concrete action is *autonomous*? The standard bioethical answer is, on the one hand, that the subject of analysis must actually perform an "action", i.e. demonstrate *intentional* behavior and, on the other hand, that this action come about in the right way. With regard to this second condition, Tom L. Beauchamp and James F. Childress (2019), for example, demand that the action in question, first, be performed by a *competent decision-maker* who, second, *understands* what is to be decided upon, and who, third, makes this decision *without any controlling influence* by other persons or any "inner constraints" due to illness. The standard model for autonomous actions thus differentiates between conditions of intent, competence, understanding, and voluntariness.

In the following, we will focus on the second component in the standard model, *the condition of competence*, since what is to be discussed here as the "triple S condition" for autonomy is commonly described in discussions of autonomy as "competence".

In order to be able to speak of a person as (sufficiently) competent to make a decision or perform an action, it is usually required that this person be (sufficiently) addressable in regard to supporting arguments and counter-arguments, with regard to her convictions, as well as to her wishes. She thus has to be in a position to arrange her wishes in proper order and to be able to envision approximately what fulfillment or frustration of her wishes would mean for her. She should also be capable of transforming her wishes into concrete "wanting" and thus to let herself initiate action – and much more. Some interpreters of autonomy, such as John Christman, demand *in addition to this* that the competence condition include the "wide variety of capacities for care, intimacy, social interaction, and the like" or that, at least, room be left for these (Christman 2011, 177). This conception is intended to take into account – as currently discussed under the catchword "relational autonomy"[1] – that personal autonomy is not only a matter of solitary self-reflection and fitness, but also the result of *interpersonal* relationships in areas of intimacy, care, or even dependency.

The following treats one particular and especially fundamental aspect of this first condition for competency that *evolves* in interpersonal relationships and is then *proven to be reliable* through them: a complex and qualified form of self-relation we sum up in the triad of self-confidence, self-assertiveness, and self-esteem. In the end, however, we show that this complex self-relation, for its part, should not be

[1] See, for example, the contributions in: Mackenzie and Stoljar 2000; critical: Ach and Schöne-Seifert 2013.

understood as a personal "competence" to be acquired and exercised. It is rather a *fundamental* ethical-existential *prerequisite* for the competence at issue here, namely, the capability for autonomous decisions and actions. In other words: this triple self-relation has little to do with our specific personal capacity for transforming our convictions, wishes, values, or intentions into corresponding actions as autonomously as possible. It has just as little to do with any skills in interaction, cooperation, or even care which are necessary in regard to interpersonal relationships. It is rather explicitly a matter of a *practical self-relation*. Or, to repeat a phrase by Paul Benson, it is not a question of "what we are capable of doing", but rather of "who we regard ourselves as being" (Benson 2000, 85).

## 4.2 Affirmation, Position, Evaluation

As previously mentioned, the fundamental self-relation for personal autonomy of action we first want to examine *conceptually* a little more closely in this section demonstrates three aspects or facets:

(a) The aspect of "self-confidence" includes not only a self-reflective, but also an *affirmative* reference to the actor's rational, motivational, imaginative, or emotional characteristics and abilities (cf. Govier 1993). If a person is supposed to be capable of autonomous decisions or actions, she has to possess not only a basic feeling for the continuity of her person, but also a fundamental "positive" sense for her own self, an elementary confidence in her most important abilities, as well as a – at least vague – feeling of her own reliability and a certain "mutuality" of her being and her actions. Anyone who, however, does *not* trust herself or her senses decisively, who thus doubts whether she can rely on her own memories, feelings, or even basic attitudes, or who faces them with distrust, is already *fundamentally* incapable of autonomy (Anderson and Honneth 2005, 134).

(b) The aspect of "self-assertiveness" goes beyond basic affirmative self-confidence and means that the person acting has a *positional* reference towards her own self. The issue here is that persons acting autonomously have to be able to be aware of their own position and also of their boundaries, and to make these limits clear, especially to other people: they take a *position*. The German word for "self-assertiveness", "Selbstbehauptung", expresses this form or facet of self-reference that makes autonomy possible very well since two things are built into it: on the one hand, self-assertiveness means that one makes an "assertion" ("Behauptung") about oneself and, in this sense, takes a position. On the other hand, it expresses that the self-positioning self raises its head ("Haupt"), so to speak, and thus takes possession of itself. Accordingly, self-assertiveness is always also a kind of self-affirmation in the form of experiencing one's own effectiveness in the world: *I* affirm *myself* through my action as the center of my actions.

(c) The aspect of elementary "self-esteem"[2] is ultimately an *evaluative* reference by the person carrying out the action towards herself. If a person is to be capable of autonomous decisions or actions, she has to consider herself "worthy" of making a (certain) decision or performing a (certain) action. She has to be able to understand herself as someone whose wishes and convictions are relevant to the impending decision or action and whose decisions or actions therefore also make a difference for her. This does not have to mean that the person should have to earn the *same respect* as all the other persons involved in regard to the impending decision or action in social or legal terms, which is a much further-reaching and nowadays customary interpretation. It is rather a basic feeling of relevance in general. To put it pointedly, it is not a question of earning moral or legal "respect", but rather, first and foremost, of not considering oneself as "nothing". If a person does not have this minimal feeling of self-esteem, she will not be in a position to relate her decisions or actions to herself in any way that is relevant *for her*. It then makes no difference – for her – whether she takes action at all or, if she does, how she decides or acts. In a certain sense, she does not even appear in these decisions or actions.

The aspects of self-confidence, self-assertiveness, and self-esteem thus refer to three forms or facets of an affirmative, positional, and evaluative reference to herself by the person taking action and are, as such, constitutive for the possibility of autonomous decision or action. In other words, for autonomous decision-making and action, a fundamental affirmation, position, and evaluation of one's own self belongs *in actu*. As will be shown below, "fundamental" means two things here: it is not only a matter of the three facets of self-relation that have to be present in at least a *minimal* manner and are especially fundamental in the sense that they have to be acquired *before* any autonomy. Additionally important is the point that the person taking action does not have to be explicitly aware of any of these forms of self-reference in the act of decision-making or taking action. Instead, it is usually the case that the person only becomes conscious of them when they purposefully direct their attention to them, for example because these self-relations are impaired or have been violated. They are, however, an important part of a person's *self-perception*, which is comprised of various forms of confirmatory self-reference, in addition to her convictions, wishes, values, and emotional inclinations.[3]

[2]This *elementary* form of self-esteem should not be confused with *more demanding* forms of qualified self-relations which are occasionally termed "self-esteem" (for example, Honneth 1996, chapter 5), but which are only realized when the (adult) person knows she is recognized as a fully adequate member of the social community.

[3]This suggestion is similar to Joel Anderson's and Axel Honneth's "recognitional account of autonomy" (Anderson and Honneth 2005; cf. Honneth 1996; Mackenzie 2000). This approach goes too far in two respects, however. Firstly, the conviction of both authors may be debatable that "full autonomy" presupposes not only fundamental self-confidence, but also moral-legal self-respect, as well as socially conveyed self-esteem, namely with regard to an ethical autonomy-ideal of the good life. It would, however, be asking too much to want this demanding self-relation to be regarded as a prerequisite for autonomous *action*. Secondly, this suggestion seems to demand that

## 4.3 The Genesis of Autonomy

Philosophy has even more difficulty in regard to genetic prerequisites for autonomous action and the question of their developmental origins. These involve presumptions about *empirical* circumstances at the beginning of human life, which are also difficult to *verify* empirically. It can find resources in developmental psychology, on the one hand, and socialization research, on the other – complicated by the fact that both of these neighboring disciplines offer anything but a uniform theoretical framework.[4] Furthermore, we must avoid interpreting these reconstructions *anthropologically* from the outset, i.e. as a reconstruction of developments in life everyone has gone through. The following considerations are valid only in social, historical, or cultural contexts for which the value of *personal autonomy* is of central importance. There may be societies in which this is not the case, even ones that are hostile towards autonomy. In such social contexts, the psychological and socialization processes that are significant for adolescents have a different nature (see, for example, Trommsdorff 1999).

With regard to contexts sympathetic to autonomy, it is debatable which "phase" of personality development should be investigated for the genetic origins of autonomy that have been summarized here for the triple S condition. Looking back, step by step, from the perspective of personal adulthood, life can be retraced – rather simplistically – through the stages of adolescence, puberty, the so-called "latent period", early childhood, and on back to infancy. Viewed in light to the three autonomy factors of affirmative self-confidence, positional self-assertiveness, and evaluative self-esteem, there may be dramatic experiences and developments in each of these phases. Moreover, it is not predetermined from the outset that all these dramatic processes of development can be dated as postnatal. The possibility must be calculated, not only in medicine but also in modern developmental psychology, research on empirical socialization, and pedagogy, that a person can also have *prenatal* influences, and that birth itself is a dramatic psychological and emotional experience that also stamps a person *perinatally* (after birth) (see Trommsdorff 1999; Janus and Haibach 1997).

Relevant literature presents three basic guiding premises concerning the genesis of competence for autonomous decisions and actions.[5] Firstly, genetic foundations for the three autonomy factors of self-confidence, self-assertiveness, and self-esteem

---

every autonomous person have "undistorted" or "non-pathological" relationships to her social environment. This would mean that persons who do *not* consider themselves integrated in such acknowledged relationships are thus not able to make any autonomous decisions, which leads to the reproach of perfectionism susceptible to paternalism.

[4] In the *psychological* respect, we will refer essentially to the psychoanalytical "object-relations theory", as well as to the tradition of "psycho-historical I-psychology" according to Erik H. Erikson. We are not able to elaborate on the tensions between these two traditions here. For an initial overview: Mitchell and Black 1995. Concerning *socialization*, we base ourselves especially on "symbolic interactionism" according to Georg H. Mead see Abels 2010.

[5] We draw primarily on classic papers: Winnicott 1965; Erikson 1977, 11.

are laid substantially in the first three years of a child's life. They may be developed further and even changed during the subsequent course of a person's life, but the respective basic prerequisites have to arise very early in life. Secondly, the formation of the self-relation outlined by these three factors is the result of typical *crises* in early childhood that cause some children to become stronger and others weaker. In each case, this depends especially upon whether and how the first reference persons for the child are successful in compensating for the ruptures experienced in the relevant crises within the childhood world by building up a confirmatory emotional structure of self-confidence, self-assertiveness and self-esteem. Thirdly, in later life, the quality and stability of self-relation depend upon the success of these infant *care* relationships, where, first of all, the relationship of the child's self to its earliest reference persons has to be taken advantage of and where the child is compensated, sometimes more, sometimes less, for ruptures experienced in its own childhood world of experiences that are absolutely necessary for its life-history. In each case, special demands arise in view of the triple S factors.

(a) The first important form of emotional confirmation the child is able to experience from others is assuring care – especially from the mother, but also from the father, siblings, or hospital staff – directly following birth (see Erikson 1977, 62ff.; cf. Leu 1999, 83f.). After a phase of complete intrauterine care, which is often described in psychological literature as a "symbiosis" between mother and child, the newborn experiences genuine social or inter-subjective care for the first time; it immediately experiences whether it can rely on other people (who, at first, are only recognizable as vague shadows).[6] The infant needs warmth, nourishment, and emotional care and attention, and getting this is a confirmation that creates trust in its protective surroundings. If the infant does *not* get this confirmation or only gets it insufficiently, for example, as the result of temporary or even permanent absence of caring reference persons, a corresponding fundamental feeling of social distrust may already prevail after a short time.[7] In *both* cases, however, the newborn experiences itself as physically and emotionally needy and dependent, but, *at the same time*, also as partially "autonomous" in the sense that it experiences itself as *different* from its surroundings. This, in turn, is a part of the experience, important for maturity processes and for later life, that temporary phases with absence of others, lack of care, "cutting the umbilical cord", and being alone are actually "survivable" (cf. Mahler et al. 1975). More and more, this also turns the often crisis-prone trust in *others* into a first form of affirmative *self-confidence* that, in the beginning, might still be based on the literally organically grown feeling that the child can trust not only its own reference persons, but also itself and the ability of its own organs to cope with its inner drives (Erikson 1977, 70).

[6] As an introduction to research on infants, still very worth reading: Dornes 1993.

[7] Trust and mistrust do not exclude each other in the world of a child since *each* child has temporary experiences of sometimes adequate and sometimes inadequate care. Psychologically decisive for the process of maturing is whether it is *fundamental* social *trust* or fundamental *mistrust* that remains.

(b) Once immediate postnatal care is fairly well ensured, the child's second experienceable form of emotional confirmation by others has to do with the recognition it demands from its reference persons that it increasingly demonstrates its "own will". Even the needy newborn's first screams can be understood as precursors of the demonstrative articulation of the child's personal will to make itself be recognized as its *own* person and thus already an "autonomous" being in specific circumstances. To some extent, the child itself is aware of its own will when it does not experience its surroundings as compliant, but rather as emotionally and materially inadequate or even resistant to its demands. Consequently, the self-reflective insight that one has an autonomous will seems to be the developmental result of repeated *frustration* of this will. Moreover, the child's demonstrative "fight" for the gratification of its needs, for example by screaming or throwing objects, increasingly becomes a "life and death" struggle (Hegel), or at least a struggle for *self-assertiveness*. The child learns to assert its will, even in face of opposition. To put this psychological situation *anatomically*, the latent *double* wish in the term "self-assertiveness" mentioned above – the wish for positional self-affirmation, on the one hand, and for ensuing self-appropriation by raising its own head, on the other – is soon expressed by the child months later when it literally begins "to stand on its own two feet". And, while the child is gaining these first experiences about its own effectiveness, the quality and stability of the self-assertiveness it has generated will, in the end, depend on whether the child's reference persons are willing not only to tolerate this early form of autonomy, but also to be noticeably affirmative towards it and recognize it.

(c) Thus, it is only when affirmative self-confidence has evolved in the first step and a just as fundamental capability for positional self-assertiveness in the second that the end result can be what has been reconstructed here as the basic genetic form of evaluative *self-esteem*. Over time, defense of one's own will on the basis of elementary self-confidence becomes leading a life that is increasingly diverse in content and also more demanding socially. Within this framework the child is not only increasingly experienced as a passive recipient of attentive benefits, but also experiences herself as an "active player" who seems to be important. After a while, the child usually does not feel alone with her need for interaction and closeness. The child's first reference persons, upon whom she may, at first, feel one-sidedly dependent, also show that they long for commitment and interchange.[8] And, in phases of temporary separation and when faced with the subsequent "joy of reunion", the child realizes not only that *other* people are of great value, but also that it is very important *for* others, too. It is this elementary appreciation that is internalized and transformed into feelings of *self-esteem* and of one's own "autonomous" relevance – a feeling based on the certainty, which cannot be taken for granted and must sometimes be sought anew, that one's own life is relevant, for oneself and for others.

[8] For the complexity of infant interaction and the child's contribution to this, see the significant work by Martin Dornes (for example, Dornes 1993, 2006).

**Table 4.1** Triple S Developmental Stages in the Child's First to Third Years[a]

| | | | | |
|---|---|---|---|---|
| *Stage 1* | SELF-CONFIDENCE | earlier forms | earlier forms | → |
| *Stage 2* | later forms | SELF-ASSERTIVENESS | earlier forms | → |
| *Stage 3* | later forms | later forms | SELF-ESTEEM | → |
| ↓ | ↓ | ↓ | ↓ | |

[a]We adopt and modify a diagram from Erikson (1977, 60)

> Accordingly, a child – and then later perhaps the adult, too – will partially lack this evaluative self-relation if she does *not* see her own relevance reflected in others (Table 4.1).[9]

Explanation of the table: Pertinent studies in developmental psychology surmise that each of the three autonomy factors develops at a different time in an infant's life (each underlain in grey), essentially as a reaction to typical biographical crises: inadequate care, obstacles, separation. In addition, it can be assumed that the three stages are necessarily built upon one another. This means that without affirmative self-confidence, there is no positional self-assertiveness, and, without this, no evaluative self-esteem. Of course, this does not mean that the three aspects come about abruptly, completely, and irrevocably in the child's development. It is rather that they are initiated ("earlier forms"), develop (underlain in grey), and then progress further ("later forms"). This marks a significant gradualism in the model that extends from preliminary stages of insufficiently developed self-relation to sufficiently developed main stages. It also means that under beneficial surrounding conditions, these self-relations "mature" (cf. the title of Winnicott 1965). Nevertheless, they remain susceptible to injuries in later life, as will be shown below.

Furthermore, the arrows at the bottom and right edge of the table signal that the three autonomy factors *after* early child development in the first 3 years may go through further stages of development (↓) and that still more fundamental aspects (→) that could be relevant for autonomous action and decision-making in these early phases of development of individual self-relation may also follow. What these might be remains unanswered here.[10] We limit ourselves to the three, in our opinion, central self-relations. Nevertheless, the basic openness of the model should be emphasized since it allows for an important second gradualism: as mentioned at the beginning, this analysis focuses on conditions for autonomous competence in decision-making and actions. However, the arrows signal that these only mark *one* end of a scale for the development of autonomy whose end is the fully developed ideal of totally autonomous *life*.[11]

[9] For the biographical consequences of disturbances in early relationships, see the groundbreaking work by John Bowlby (for example, Bowlby 1982).

[10] Consideration should be given to whether moral or even motor abilities are also important for the genesis of the capability for autonomous action, for example.

[11] See also the eight-step model for "psycho-historical development": Erikson 1977.

## 4.4 The Vulnerability of Autonomy

The genetic triple S stages are accompanied by typical susceptibilities and vulnerabilities that continue at least partially in later life and then – from a socio-philosophical viewpoint – will, in certain cases, have an effect as social "pathologies" of autonomy, as they are sometimes termed in socio-philosophical recognition theory.[12] When viewing the obvious parallels between the history of genetic development, on the one hand, and the later course of life, on the other, recognition theory admittedly tends to overlook the *relative independence* of the two. There may be good reasons for the view that a person may be more immune to injuries to her autonomy in later life the more extensively she has experienced recognition in earliest childhood. Exactly the opposite could also be true: the less self-confidence, self-assertiveness, and self-esteem developed in earliest childhood, the more susceptible the interplay between autonomy and commitment for an adult in view of the recognition denied her.[13] However, a person who has grown up with very *little* self-confidence, self-assertiveness, and self-esteem is not "lost", in the sense that these early deficits cannot be compensated for in later life. Nor is a child with very *pronounced* triple S factors completely immune from dramatic feelings of insecurity in later life. However, the three basic autonomy factors prove to be a "foundation" in the sense that the respective convulsions have to be *fundamental*. In the following, we focus on convulsions that result from problematic or even pathologically distorted relationships to others.[14]

(a) As stated above, a person's elementary *self-confidence* is based on the feeling of being able to rely especially on her own body and its most important functions, as well as on her own senses. Since this self-confidence is genetically the result of reflection on the trust a person has built up and placed in her first reference persons and in their qualities of care and protection, inter-subjective injuries to self-confidence often assail this spot in later life – interpersonal encroachments or assaults[15] that cause the person, who feels confident that others have a fundamentally peaceful, friendly, or even loving attitude, to lose fundamentally the feeling of being able to rely on herself, her own body, her abilities, or even her own thinking processes. Since the *deepest* layer of practical self-relation is affected, the aggression or invasive harm is often

---

[12] For clarification of the socio-philosophical term in pathology in connection with Axel Honneth, see: Pollmann 2005, 30–37.

[13] See the fascinating analysis: Benjamin 1988.

[14] There are also *non-social* adversities, for example, the failure of great hopes or a serious illness. However, we blank out any non-social negative experiences since we want to indicate the extent to which these thoughts have normative or moral consequences and that moral consequences are only the result if other people are involved in a demanding or hurtful way.

[15] "Encroachments" or "assaults" on a person do not at all necessarily lead to partial or complete loss of triple S factors. Whether this loss comes about depends greatly on how stable the self-relation concerned is. Consequently, the more stable a self-relation is, the graver, more far-reaching, and more aggressive the offence has to be if the person suffers lasting damage.

correspondingly grave and occurs rather seldom, as in cases of physical violence, sexual abuse, rape, or torture, and even gross negligence, isolation, or brain-washing practices.[16]

(b) The aspect of fundamental *self-assertiveness*, on the other hand, comes from the developmental fact that the small child who is frustrated in her needs increasingly feels a gap between her will and the often resistant will of others. Later life holds numerous such frustrations that will compel the person concerned to resist the will of others and, if necessary, implement her will despite opposition. This self-assertiveness may be successful or may fail at times, and compromises will often have to be made. In order for self-assertiveness to be fundamentally *impossible*, other people have to take away, in a very basic way, any chance of one's asserting one's own will and seeing one's own personal function confirmed (or at least tolerated) in the social surroundings. This could come from invasive encroachments or immoral behavior that leave fundamental doubts about the existence of one's *own* will (which it would be important to assert), or at least make it difficult to continue to exist with one's "head held high": compulsion and coercion, instrumentalization and exploitation, but also acts of indignity, abasement, and humiliation.[17]

(c) Finally, the aspect of fundamental *self-esteem* has been interpreted here as the developmental result or incorporation of intersubjectively conveyed awareness that one is not only dependent upon other people, but also has significant worth for at least some of these others. Consequently, the practical certainty sets in of individual but also social relevance in life that will later support one existentially, but can also be convulsed in later life if someone gives the person the feeling of being "nothing" of any importance. This is especially the case in situations and through unsocial practices whereby someone not only contests that the person has the *same* moral or legal worth as any other human being, but denies her *any* value as a human (see, for example, Margalit 1996). In such a case, the complete deprivation of evaluative relevance is accompanied by the danger of incorporating this experience into a feeling of one's own irrelevance or inferiority. Some examples of forms of unsocial behavior showing this tendency are demonstrative forms of ignoring or failing to notice a person, social exclusion, the deprivation of liberty, and especially also severe forms of mobbing, disregard, or discrimination.[18]

The complex relationship between conditions for susceptibility to injury in later life linked with the triple S factors is illustrated in the following table, which should be interpreted as follows: once the three central self-relations of self-confidence, self-assertiveness, and self-esteem have been roughly established in infancy, they result in three "deep layers" of practical self-relations, one on top of the other. This means, on the one hand, that an injury to deeper layers can "break through" to the layers

[16] See the analyses oriented on phenomena: Scarry 1987; Sofsky 1996.

[17] See the relevant articles in: Pollmann 2010.

[18] See also articles in: Pollmann 2010.

**Table 4.2** Triple S Susceptibility in Later Life

| | *Dramatic losses* →↓ | | |
|---|---|---|---|
| *Deep layer 1* | SELF-CONFIDENCE | →↓ | |
| *Deep layer 2* | ↑← | SELF-ASSERTIVENESS | →↓ |
| *Deep layer 3* | | ↑← | SELF-ESTEEM |
| | ↑← *Increasing invasiveness* | | |

above (→↓). It also means, on the other hand, that invasive encroachments on external self-relations with others have an even more serious effect the deeper they penetrate into that external self-relation with someone else (↑←) (Table 4.2).

## 4.5 Conclusion

Among the elementary competences a person has to have in order to be capable of autonomous decision-making and action, there is the triad of self-confidence, self-assertiveness, and self-esteem, in addition to various rational and social abilities. These self-relations are formed and developed in interactive childhood relationships, especially in intimate family relationships with material and emotional care and attention. Relevant reconstructions make it questionable, however, whether it is actually a matter of acquiring corresponding "competences" in regard to these three self-relations, as bioethical discussion seems to suggest. On the one hand, the triple S factors prove to be so fundamental in the history of a person's life that they should rather be understood as an existentially indispensable *basic prerequisite* of the ability to make decisions and perform actions autonomously (and thus not as a triple competence). Moreover, the term competence suggests that the abilities in question can be acquired, learned, and practiced individually. However, this typical assumption seems to be misleading for the triad of self-confidence, self-assertiveness, and self-esteem, at least from a genetic perspective, when it is a question of early childhood acquisition of this triple self-relation or its failure. In view of the early developmental history of a person, it must be concluded that the very first self-relation that should be acquired in partially "unavailable" relationships supplying love and care may be unavailable to the persons concerned and their reference persons. This means that it is a question of biographical "fate" whether a child gets the care and attention she needs very early in order to be able to make decisions and perform actions autonomously in later life.

Even if we have spoken of only the *descriptive* criteria for autonomous actions in this contribution, some *normative* conclusions can nevertheless be drawn from our observations. Whoever, for whatever reasons and in whatever way, is interested in assuring that persons are capable of autonomous decisions or actions will, firstly, have to ensure that they are able to grow up in more or less intact social relationships and experience more or less intact intimate relationships. It is evident that this insight would have far-reaching social, political, cultural, and even pedagogical consequences. This would, however, be the normative aspiration that follows from our *genetic* analysis. Furthermore, whoever, for whatever reasons and in whatever way, is interested in assuring that persons are capable of autonomous decisions or actions will, secondly, have to ensure that the triad of self-confidence, self-assertiveness, and self-esteem is not infringed upon or even destroyed through (systematic) invasive encroachments or unsocial practices in later life. This is the normative aspiration that follows from the *socio-philosophical* perspective of our observations. The reason for this double aspiration is that more or less intact intimate and social relationships are indispensable not only for *acquiring* a self-relation enabling autonomy, but also for *preserving* it later, which means that the demand for absence and abolition of certain forms of destructive social relationships is normatively urgent in both respects.

**Conflict of Interest** The authors state that there are no conflicts of interest.

## References


Abels, H. 2010. *Interaktion, Identität, Präsentation*. 5th ed. Opladen: Verlag für Sozialwissenschaften.

Ach, J.S., and B. Schöne-Seifert. 2013. "Relationale Autonomie"– Eine kritische Analyse. In *Patientenautonomie. Theoretische Grundlagen – Praktische Anwendungen*, ed. C. Wiesemann and A. Simon, 42–60. Münster: Mentis.

Anderson, J., and A. Honneth. 2005. Autonomy, Vulnerability, Recognition, and Justice. In *Autonomy and the Challenges to Liberalism*, ed. J. Christman and J. Anderson, 127–149. New York/Cambridge: Cambridge University Press.

Beauchamp, T.L., and J.F. Childress. 2019. *Principles of Biomedical Ethics*. 8th ed. Oxford: Oxford University Press.

Benjamin, J. 1988. *Bonds of Love*. New York: Pantheon Books.

Benson, P. 2000. Feeling Crazy: Self-Worth and the Social Character of Responsibility. In *Relational Autonomy*, ed. C. Mackenzie and N. Stoljar, 72–93. Oxford/New York: Oxford University Press.

Bowlby, J. 1982. *Attachment and Loss*. 2nd ed. New York: Basic Books.

Christman, J. 2011. *The Politics of Persons*. Cambridge: Cambridge University Press.

Dornes, M. 1993. *Der kompetente Säugling*. Frankfurt a.M.: Fischer.

———. 2006. *Die Seele des Kindes*. Frankfurt a.M.: Fischer.

Erikson, E.H. 1977. Wachstum und Krisen der gesunden Persönlichkeit. In *E. H. Erikson: Identität und Lebenszyklus*, 55–122. Frankfurt a.M: Suhrkamp.

Govier, T. 1993. Self-Trust, Autonomy, and Self-Esteem. *Hypatia* 8 (1): 99–120.

Honneth, A. 1996. *Struggle for Recognition*. Cambridge: MIT Press.

Janus, L., and S. Haibach, eds. 1997. *Seelisches Erleben vor und während der Geburt*. Neu-Isenburg: LinguaMed.

Leu, H.R. 1999. Die "biographische Situation" als Bezugspunkt eines sozialisationstheoretischen Subjektverständnisses. In *Zwischen Autonomie und Verbundenheit*, ed. L. Krappmann and H.R. Leu, 77–107. Frankfurt a.M: Suhrkamp.
Mackenzie, C. 2000. Imagining Oneself Otherwise. In *Relational Autonomy*, ed. C. Mackenzie and N. Stoljar, 124–150. Oxford/New York: Oxford University Press.
Mackenzie, C., and N. Stoljar, eds. 2000. *Relational Autonomy*. Oxford/New York: Oxford University Press.
Mahler M.S., Pine F., and Bergman A., eds. 1975. *The Psychological Birth of the Human Infant: Symbiosis and Individuation*. New York: Basic Books.
Margalit, A. 1996. *Decent Society*. Cambridge: Harvard Univ. Press.
Mitchell, S.A., and M.J. Black. 1995. *Freud and Beyond: A History of Modern Psychoanalytic Thought*. New York: Basic Books.
Pollmann, A. 2005. *Integrität*. Bielefeld: Transcript.
———. 2010. *Unmoral. Ein philosophisches Handbuch*. München: C.H. Beck.
Scarry, E. 1987. *The Body in Pain: The Making and Unmaking of the World*. Oxford: Oxford University Press.
Sofsky, W. 1996. *Traktat über die Gewalt*. Frankfurt a.M.: Fischer.
Trommsdorff, G. 1999. Autonomie und Verbundenheit im kulturellen Vergleich von Sozialisationsbedingungen. In *Zwischen Autonomie und Verbundenheit*, ed. L. Krappmann and H.R. Leu, 392–419. Frankfurt a.M: Suhrkamp.
Winnicott, D.W. 1965. *Maturational Processes and the Facilitating Environment*. New York: International Universities Press.

# Chapter 5
# Autonomy, Respect, and Joint Deliberation

**John Christman**

**Abstract** Respecting the autonomy of agents grounds various obligations to others such as non-interference, deference to her authority over self-regarding decisions, limitations on paternalism, and so on. According to a broadly liberal moral sensibility, respecting others in this way implies accepting (in some sense) the values they autonomously hold even if they are judged problematic, immoral, self-destructive, or otherwise non-ideal. In discussions of such respect, it is generally assumed that persons expressing that respect (or not) have no direct bearing on whether the subject of that respect is herself autonomous. However, in many situations, persons interact in a way that helps establish or re-establish the autonomy of one or both of these agents themselves.

For example, the would-be paternalist may be a therapist whose professional obligation is to facilitate the process of re-establishing autonomy for vulnerable victims of trauma. In such scenarios, the usual lines between hard and soft paternalism, as well as the standard liberal rejection of the former, do not apply. Still, it would be wrong for the aid worker to simply impose her views of a decent life on the struggling person. How, then, do we reformulate restrictions on paternalism and other such normative strictures grounded in respect for autonomy in scenarios where the relationship between client and aid worker is itself a crucial part of the process that results in the self-governing agency of the client?

This paper explores these issues and argues that such (very typical) scenarios indicate that conceptions of autonomy must view the self as diachronic as well as socially constituted but also must be sensitive to the ways that autonomy can sometimes be (re-)established only with others' help. In particular, the obligation to remain relatively neutral toward the content of others' values in showing respect for their autonomy (the broad liberal sensibility) must be reformulated to take into account the way interpersonal dynamics themselves help establish the autonomy with which persons hold the values that they hold. These observations are applied to certain cases of aid and care where such questions are central.

J. Christman (✉)
Philosophy, Political Science, and Women's Studies, Penn State University, University Park, PA, USA
e-mail: jpc11@psu.edu



J. F. Childress, M. Quante (eds.), *Thick (Concepts of) Autonomy*, Philosophical Studies Series 146, https://doi.org/10.1007/978-3-030-80991-1_5

## 5.1 Autonomy, Respect, and Joint Deliberation

The moral demand that we respect the autonomy of other agents grounds various obligations to others such as those regarding non-interference, deference to their authority over self-regarding decisions, limitations on paternalism, and so on. According to a broadly liberal moral sensibility, respecting others in this way implies accepting (in some sense) the values they autonomously hold even if they are judged to be problematic, immoral, self-destructive, or otherwise non-ideal. However, in discussions of such respect, it is generally assumed that persons expressing that respect (or not) act and reflect independently of the object of respect. But in many situations, persons interact in a way that helps establish or re-establish the autonomy of one or both of these agents together or which partly constitutes the exercise of their autonomy.[1]

For example, two romantic partners are considering whether to have children or not. Such a choice has profound implications for each of their lives, but their commitment to each other means that they want the decision and the reasoning going into it to be mutual and collaborative. Both rest on their values and self-defining commitments as separate individuals but also allow their thinking to be shaped by their interaction and mutual commitment. Certainly this commitment and associated trust would be violated if one of the partners engaged in manipulation in order to get the other to come to his way of thinking. The obligation to respect the wishes and perspective of the other would be violated.

Another example might be an aid worker or therapist whose professional obligation is to facilitate the process of re-establishing autonomy for vulnerable victims of trauma. In such scenarios, the standard liberal principle to respect the autonomy of others in their decisions is based on the obligation to respect the person's wishes if she is autonomous or to treat her with care and benevolence if she is not. But in either case it would be wrong for the aid worker to simply impose her views of a decent life onto the struggling person. How, then, do we reformulate restrictions on paternalism and other obligations grounded in respect for autonomy in scenarios where the relationship between one person and another is itself a crucial part of the dynamic by which the autonomy of one or both of them is established or exercised?

What further complicates this issue is that while autonomy has traditionally been thought to apply paradigmatically to individuals considered in themselves, without essential reference to relations with others, that presumption has been rejected recently in theories of autonomy that either see that property as essentially relational or as applying to persons understood as constituted by social and interpersonal relations. In the situations being imagined here, however, the deliberating partners are engaged in actions that either help establish or help the exercise of the other partner's autonomy by way of their specific interaction. The problem is how each person can show respect for the autonomy of that other in such intertwined situations.

---

[1] I have discussed similar issues in Christman 2014a.

In what follows, I want to lay out the problem as I see it and propose (guardedly) a solution. I will proceed by first sketching the broad outlines of a view of autonomy that sees it as a trait applying to individuals but which nevertheless contains elements that relate to the social and relational dynamics between persons. I will also outline what I mean by the "liberal sensibility", meaning a set of *pro tanto* duties to defer to the values of others out of respect for their autonomy.[2] In Section III, I will describe what I call "partnerships" where the interpersonal dynamics of two individuals have a causal and constitutive relation to the establishment or exercise of autonomy of one or both of them. I will then describe how such partnerships pose a challenge for the liberal sensibility I mentioned. In the closing section I will suggest a set of guidelines for interpersonal respect in such situations which reflects the requirements of autonomy (as I have described it) and remains faithful to the liberal sensibility by which we generally express respect for one another. My overall conclusion is that the obligation to show respect for another's autonomy remains in force in such partnerships but must be reformulated to take into account the way that interpersonal dynamics themselves help establish the autonomy with which persons hold the values that they hold. Such a conclusion implies, in turn, that we see autonomy as not only socially structured but extended over time.

## 5.2 The General Contours of Autonomy

In order to consider the demand that we respect others' autonomy we need to look closely at the idea of autonomy itself. As we will see, that idea is hardly a simple one and its particular components will operate differently in the mechanics of cooperative deliberation of the sort we will consider. To get clear on those operations, let us take a brief overview of the standard contemporary understandings of the idea of autonomy that populate the recent literature.

Autonomy can refer to particular decisions or to the status of the person generally. Autonomy can also be seen as a matter of degree or as a threshold property. Insofar as autonomy marks the aspect of persons by which moral respect is grounded, then it must be seen as an all or nothing affair, at least insofar as prescriptions of this sort of respect do not vary in degree. Moreover, in cases of interest here, the respect in question regards major decisions that rest on the person's most basic value scheme, in respect of which the person's autonomy is in question.

Standard approaches to autonomy see that characteristic as the ability of the person to guide her life from her own perspective rather than be manipulated by others or be forced into a particular path by surreptitious forces. Conditions for autonomy in this sense have typically included what have been called competency

[2] As I will explain, the phrase "defer to" does not mean one must abide by or follow others' values, but the posture I refer to here includes obligations to pay special heed to others' desires and values in some way (which may include not interfering with their pursuit of them even when one thinks they are wrong-headed).

conditions, on the one hand, and authenticity conditions, on the other. The former refer to the agent's ability to form intentions and engage in action voluntarily, and with sufficient information. These conditions may also include requirements of rationality, motivational competence, self-control, emotional stability, and other conditions.

More complex are the requirements of what is here called "authenticity". Requirements of authenticity attempt to determine when the values, desires, character traits, and so on that orient a person's choices and move her to action are truly her own in a way that coincides with the idea of self-government. Those who are acting competently but on the basis of values that they have been forced or manipulated into adopting, or which arise out of pathological, oppressive, or overly constraining conditions, are not acting as self-governing agents. Various accounts of this set of conditions have been given. For example, many follow Harry Frankfurt and Gerald Dworkin in requiring that the person be able to critically reflect on her first level motives and accept them as her own or in keeping with her deepest cares.[3] Lack of autonomy can stem from many conditions on this model then. Compulsion, temporary or protracted mental disability, and addiction are most often mentioned as examples, as are brainwashing and manipulation of the psychic economy of the agent. These conditions undercut the person's ability to reflectively accept her first-order motives and/or the way that she has come to develop them.

However, it has been claimed that such a view assumes an overly individualistic understanding of agency and value. For example, those whose self-conception makes reference to a cultural, religious, or social role but who are permanently removed from the conditions in which such a role can be exercised, may lack the capacity for self-governing agency, and not simply because of a lack of a capacity as an individual. The goals in question may no longer make sense in the new conditions because the social interactions that gave them meaning no longer take place. The person's practical identity by which he or she considers options, makes plans and considers questions of value is completely fractured because of this social breakdown.[4]

There are also many different accounts of the role of social interaction for autonomy. On my own view I have tried to stress the socio-historical nature of the *self* who is doing the reflecting and the social nature of many of the values and commitments that are the object of that reflection. Additionally, I stress how the autonomous person must accept her values and motives (and other life conditions) as part of an ongoing historical self-narrative, so that autonomy must be seen as diachronic in these ways. Hence, a person is autonomous if she can reflectively accept her condition in light of its history and ongoing narrative and do so without deep

[3] See Frankfurt 1987 and 1992 and Dworkin 1989.

[4] Jonathan Lear examines the case of Plenty Coups, the leader of the Crow Indian nation in the U.S. whose traditional tribal way of life had been completely destroyed. On Lear's analysis, Plenty Coups's values, motives and social self-understanding was thereby fractured, making him unable to find a way forward until he was able to reconstruct a sense of social identity in a new setting. See Lear 2006

self-alienation, given her social situation.[5] Others have insisted that others' recognition of the person's normative authority or ability to answer for herself be part of the social conditions of autonomy.[6]

So for now let us say that the central test for autonomy that I favor (omitting many details) is that the autonomous person is such that she is disposed to reflectively accept her motives (or other features of herself relevant to action) without alienation in light of her history and social condition as part of an ongoing personal self-narrative. This dispositional reflective self-acceptance is meant to help avoid the problems of regress or groundlessness raised against standard hierarchical models of autonomy where second-order reflection plays a crucial endorsing role for first-order attitudes and motives. On my view, these problems are avoided insofar as these reflections arise out of the agent's diachronic practical identity, the broad and deep set of evaluative structures that orient judgment for the person. This borrows language from Christine Korsgaard but is also akin to what Frankfurt refers to as our deepest cares and what Michael Bratman refers to as our self-defining projects (Frankfurt 1999; Korsgaard 1996; Bratman 2007, ch. 2).

Also, however, my view accepts the idea that much intentional, self-governing action is not guided by *actual* reflection. Many such actions are habitual, automatic, or arising from such strongly held convictions where consideration of doing otherwise might be "unthinkable" for the person, in Frankfurt's phrase. The reflective test I use here is dispositional and involves various additional requirements ensuring that the reflection in question adequately expresses the viewpoint and evaluative orientation of the agent.[7] I will return to this point.

Indeed, intentional self-governing action on my view merely involves what we can call reflective self-monitoring: this is the function of passive acceptance of the motives that guide action but with a disposition to "step in" as it were if things go awry. Like a driver whose mind wanders, one is still in control of oneself because one is able to snap into concentration and change one's direction or speed if the occasion called for it. I call such self-monitoring "reflective" only in the sense that the person is in a position to give reasons for her habitual action if asked. The reflection need not be "deep" in the sense of bringing into question the very value formation that defines her as an agent (her practical identity), but the person is able to give an account to others if asked under appropriate conditions.[8] That is to say, the person must be able to give reasons that reflect her practical identity and which, in turn, reflexively affirms her commitment to that identity. Such reflective reasoning, of course, may come to an end in statements like "that is the way I am" but they must also express statements of the form "and that is a worthwhile way to be".

---

[5] See Christman 2009.

[6] See, e.g., Mackenzie 2008, Westlund 2003, Anderson and Honneth 2005, Oshana 2006, Benson 2005, and Christman and Anderson 2005.

[7] See Christman 2009, chap. 7.

[8] This is to borrow the requirement of "answerability" stressed by writers such as Andrea Westlund and Paul Benson. See Benson 2005 and Westlund 2003.

That is to say, one accepts oneself without alienation in my sense when one thinks one's motives are worth having – that they are coherent and at least minimally justified from one's own point of view – and that they feel intelligible *as one's own*. The addict, the mentally impaired person, and the deeply conflicted agent does not sense her values as worth having as her own in this way. The motives that spur action for such a person are not ones that she can see as giving her reasons to continue so acting. In this way, she is alienated in my sense.

Being (self-) alienated means feeling and judging one's motives to be in such conflict (with each other or with other deeper self-defining values) that their self-justificational force is undercut (relative to an alternative condition one can imagine), even if they in the end move one to act. The alienated person also will not experience the appropriate affective and emotional concomitants to decisions, such as pride and shame, in the right way. This sense of self-fragmentation is important for it marks a lack of autonomy but is described in a way that does not postulate a separated and disembodied point of view from which the person judges her identity and condition. The assumption that such a completely detached point of view is available and psychologically operative has been rightly criticized as untenable.[9]

Much more can be said about the details of this and other models of autonomy, and we will return to some of these issues presently. For now, let us turn to the broad requirement of interpersonal respect required of moral agents and how such respect is complicated by acknowledging the way in which people often deliberate in close interaction with others, making both the development and exercise of autonomy – the object of such respect – dependent on that very interaction.

## 5.3 The Liberal Sensibility

It is no accident that in calling this perspective the "liberal" sensibility I utilize a political notion, as the ethical principles I will refer to arise from the moral and political framework of modernist liberal social philosophy. But the ideas I mention here are neither inherently political nor reliant on those broader commitments. I want only give a name to a cluster of what I hope are uncontroversial ethical prescriptions that apply to interpersonal relations and involve acknowledgement of the moral importance others' autonomy.

Respect for others as autonomous beings is a fundamental part of the common sense moral obligations structuring everyday social life. One need not be a Kantian to accept the idea that others' capacity to make self-governing decisions serves as the object of value and respect in our interactions with them, even if obligations of respect of this sort might be grounded in some broader moral framework (such as utilitarianism or virtue).

[9] See, e.g., Sandel 1982.

All I want to identify here is a set of *pro tanto* obligations that figure in some central way in the ethical principles with which we deal with each other, even if such obligations are often overridden or in competition with other quite different considerations. But insofar as respect for autonomy has this central ethical role, it has a certain structure that should be identified. Respect for autonomy grounds various obligations of non-interference, limitations on paternalism, deference to others' authority in matters relating to them, conferral of equal status to such persons in contexts of collective deliberation, tolerating those we disapprove of, letting people have their say, and other such obligations. In these ways, in interpersonal relations, one person's desire to advance her own interests or the interests of the persons she encounters must take seriously into account or be strictly constrained by respect for the autonomous agency of those others.

In close relations between co-deliberators of the sort we will discuss in a moment, it may seem that respect for autonomy plays no role in the ethical considerations guiding the interaction, as considerations of care, love, concern and cooperation dominate the ethical scene. However, as I will emphasize, even in such relatively intimate settings, it is clear how the directive to respect one's partner as a person who is able to make up her own mind, exercise her own unique point of view, and so on, still operates at least as a background obligation framing the interaction. Caring for another can go awry, morally, if one fails to treat her also as a person who is able to competently and authentically formulate and act upon values of her own, at least when she meets the standards of autonomy we are discussing.

I hope so much is uncontroversial. The point of articulating these obligations is that they have as their object the actual capacity of persons to be self-governing. That is, insofar as others are autonomous, we owe them the treatment these obligations describe, to some significant degree. If they are not, such obligations of respect are suspended in favor of alternative moral postures, such as duties of care whose object is advancing well-being, full stop. But those ethical considerations are separable from the obligations to respect autonomy and the judgments a person makes about her own well-being she makes as an autonomous being.

While commonplace, this set of ethical strictures also presupposes a certain interpersonal dynamic that will be crucial for the problems we are discussing, namely that the person who bears the obligation to show respect in question is not typically in any way involved in the *constitution* or *exercise* of the autonomy of the person so respected. This, as we will see, is the crux of the difficulty we will be examining.

## 5.4 Partnerships

Recall that in the general schema for autonomous agency I rely on here, a person acts for motives that are her own when she competently and reflectively accepts them as part of an ongoing autobiographical narrative. Such a schema is meant to be "content neutral" in the sense that no direct reference is made to the kinds of motives or values that an autonomous person must have to count as such. Though it may well be that various particular values will be incompatible with reflective self-acceptance because of the social-psychological effects of having those values on the competence and reflective capacities of the agent, but not because of the status of those values in themselves.[10]

Also, the schema in no way assumes that the motives and values that move an agent were originally chosen by her or that they are under her control in a narrow sense. So a person may be autonomous on these models even if the entirely inherited her values and is not in a current position to alter them, psychologically speaking (what Al Mele describes as "unsheddable" values) (Mele 1995, 153–73). As long as she meets the conditions of reflective self-acceptance (with all other requirements intact), these factors will not negate her self-government.

And while the reflection in question is from the individual's point of view, there are many conditions where close interaction between people directly and indirectly determines the content and strength of the motives a person finds herself with. For example, long-term romantic partners may well see many decisions as fully collaborative ones, as I mentioned earlier, where each considers the other's needs and judgment not as a separable datum that must be weighed in balanced consideration of her own desires but very much as part of the content of those very desires. In many such cases, what we can call "cooperative reflection" takes place, where each individual considers her values and options in close interaction with the other, either in actual dialogue or in deep consideration of the other's perspective as part of one's own self-appraisal. What "I" think becomes very much constituted by what "we" think.

To give a more precise account of the interpersonal dynamics of partnerships, and for the special challenges they raise for the principle of respect for autonomy, let us briefly examine Michael Bratman's account of shared agency and, in particular, shared deliberation. For Bratman, agents have shared cooperative intentions when "each agent intends that the group perform [the] joint action in accordance with sub-plans (of the intention to perform the joint action) that mesh..."[11] By "meshing" Bratman means that the particular elements of each person's plan coheres and compliments the corresponding elements in the other's (sub-) plan. In this way, they display interlocking and reflexive intentions. They are also mutually responsive to the norms generated by their meshing (sub-)plans, for plans are hierarchically organized desires that are grounded in the past and extend into the future and carry with them directives to treat as a reason particular desires that form part of the plan. In this way, plans are normative for the people whose plans they are. Further, these intentional dynamics are commonly believed by the group members to be persisting (Bratman 2014, ch. 3).

---

[10] This is to accept, in part, what Kristinsson calls a "weakly substantive" account of autonomy. See Kristinsson 2000.

[11] Bratman 2007, 232.

In this way, what Bratman calls "modest sociality" obtains when there is mutual responsiveness on the part of participants: their shared intentions lead to their actions by way of commonly known mutual responsiveness (to shared norms) that tracks the ends they each mutually intend (Bratman 2014, ch. 4). Of greater interest to us here is how he applies this account of shared intentions to act to a view of shared *deliberation*. For the kinds of partnerships we are considering involve mutually accepted plans to deliberate together and to allow such thinking together to reflect complex interdependence. The question such phenomena gives rise to is how the autonomy of each can be maintained with such mutual interdependence and, more pointedly, how each can maintain an attitude of respect for the autonomy of the other when the reflection they mutually engage in partly constitutes that autonomy.

For Bratman, shared deliberation involves three elements: embeddedness of the shared intentions of the group, meaning that the intentions of the two (or more) agents are intentionally co-mingled; common ground of shared commitments, meaning that certain considerations that matter to us matter to other group members (our partner, say); and shared commitment to "weights", meaning a shared commitment to take certain normative considerations into account together in our deliberations. This last element is perhaps the most important and we will come back to it presently. The overall picture is that groups count as deliberating together when group members share an intention to deliberate interactively in these ways and mutually follow certain norms implicit in their guiding sub-plans and shared intentions.

Mutually committing ourselves to "weights" involves allowing ourselves to be guided by various exclusionary reasons (what counts as a default position in our reasoning, for example, or what counts as a defeater to such a position, and so on). However, mutually allowing ourselves to be guided together by the weight of these norms does not involve *valuing* the objects of such norms, Bratman argues (2014, 136–7). This is crucial, in that it means that I can deliberate together with you and in so doing let myself be guided by the common normative considerations that structure our common thinking, but in doing this I don't have to hold an independent judgment that the things such norms point to as values are values to me outside of our relationship.

An example might help: my partner and I deliberate together about whether to both accept a new academic position. In doing so we implicitly allow ourselves to be moved by certain considerations that are embedded in certain aspects of our shared plans, such as only taking a job with a salary that matches our current one. I am happy to use this consideration in our deliberation together, but it may well be the case that I don't much care about money, and I'd be happy to take a cut in salary for the new job. But I realize that doing this unilaterally will upset a certain balance in our mutual standing in negotiating as partners (if I took a cut, it would put pressure on my partner to do so and I know this would make her uncomfortable, etc.). I don't value the object of our shared normative commitment but I'm happy to be guided by it as constitutive of our agreement to think about this together.

This means that shared deliberation is compatible with interpersonal value pluralism. Two people who (when thinking independently) have different values can be guided by norms that presuppose such values as a constraint on their co-thinking. We need this shared policy about weights to ensure the reliability, predictability, and intelligibility of our deliberations, but we can commit to such a policy for divergent reasons. Our shared commitment to these weights is based in part on the reasons we have for our partnership to begin with (for Bratman our sociality). Valuing this sociality may be based on its desirability, its feasibility or on some obligation we have to do so (Bratman 2014, 144). But in any case, we value the partnership and the shared deliberations that go with it in ways that give us reasons to shape our thinking in particular ways that we wouldn't have if reasoning alone.

Bratman claims that such shared deliberation and activity can express the autonomy of the group so acting (2014, chap. 6). However, this view of collective agency is something I want to put to the side for now, for my worry is not how the partnership acts as a kind of autonomous agent but how the respective partners maintain their autonomy as individuals even if engaged in such an intimate deliberative interaction. This is necessary so we can ask our question about respect.

But the example of long-term partners I just gave suggests relative equality of power, at least as I am describing it (perhaps in a naively idealized tone). Such partnerships can be labeled SP partnerships, for "symmetrical power" partnerships. Also of importance in this context are those partnership connections where one person's judgment and values has a constitutive and causal relation to a second person's deliberative perspective about an important decision but not vice versa. An aid worker, therapist, physician, or care-giver might occupy this position relative to an extremely vulnerable or needful client. These will be labeled asymmetrical power (AP) partnerships.

Although the question of mutual respect for autonomy can be raised about partnerships of any type of power configuration, it has particular poignancy when asked about partnerships of asymmetrical power, in particular those where the relatively less powerful person is in a fragile and vulnerable position. The dimensions of power operating in such situations are numerous, and may include differences in intelligence, social status, resources, authority, and so on. All of these are relevant to real-world cases. But for the theoretical purposes at hand, I want to focus on the way that the judgments and actions of the one person can affect and in a way help constitute the reflective deliberations of the subject. In such a situation, I will argue, the "liberal sensibility" we discussed earlier will be complicated, to say the least.

Consider a vulnerable and struggling young woman, Christina, who has just been traumatized because of being forced into sex work. Imagine she has been "rescued" from such a condition in a foreign country.[12] This coercive sex work forced Christina to engage in activities that dramatically violated the self-defining value orientation of her earlier life. In addition to the substandard conditions of her life as a sex worker, this work involved trauma and violence that Christina must now work to

[12] I discuss a similar example in 2014a.

recover from. A social worker is working with her to determine, for example, what her options are regarding such things as whether to return home or remain in the destination country (where she is highly vulnerable to either being forced or "choosing" to return to prostitution). After medical, nutritional, and housing resources are secured for Christina, a therapeutic process begins where the social worker helps her gain a sense of confidence and psychological (and material) capacity to make such decisions about her life.

Christina's vulnerability here is pronounced, as is her dependence on the judgment and actions of the social worker (call her Seba). Many people in Christina's situation return to the life of prostitution (and drugs) both out of fear of returning home, where they may face shame and rejection, but also as a possible mode of survival in a context of few feasible options. Such people can put themselves in a position, however, to engage in prostitution in ways that allow them to survive and even send funds back to their families as remittances, even if such activity continues to involve extreme risk.

Consider further that Christina was brought up in a religious setting that was built around the virtues of sexual modesty. Her practical identity – the virtues and obligations she regarded herself as defined by – structured the sense of her future and memories of her past. However, after the experience of forced sex work, she can no longer embrace that identity in its original form. The fact that her family and home community would not accept her because of this drives home this point in tragic detail.

In Christina's case the aid worker must engage in the process of therapy in ways that delicately negotiates a process of both recovering from trauma but also forming a renegotiated practical identity that will contain value commitments relating to self-respect, dignity, and perhaps religious obligation.[13] The social worker, of course, has tremendous influence over the course of this renegotiation of Christina's sense of herself. She might have to decide, for example, whether to counsel Christina away from considering any options that might lead her back to prostitution or other risky activities. In doing so, should she judge it best, Seba would be influencing strongly the value orientation that Christina develops over the course of treatment.

In addition, the process of Christina's regaining the competencies that are required of autonomy is subtly guided by Seba's therapeutic attentions. Christina's goal, we can assume, is both to settle on a life plan that is realistic and attainable for her, given her situation, and to do so in ways that she can live with as her own, so to regain her autonomy relative to such goals. Seba's role, then, is to aid this process cooperatively with Christina but in ways that make the outcome Christina's own.

Such scenarios are sadly common. I simplify here grossly in order to focus on the (for us) central normative issue at play, namely what strictures on paternalistic interventions are applicable here based on respect for the (perhaps nascent) autonomy of the subject. Clearly questions surrounding Christina's competence, rationality, mental health, and so on are relevant here. But what is not often noted in discussions of similar cases, is that the judgments and actions of the aid worker herself are also highly relevant to whether the woman is autonomous.

[13] For a sensitive and insightful discussion of recovery from trauma in this way, see Brison 2003.

Again, I simplify here by considering a dyadic relation between two persons, while in fact cases of this sort will involve complex networks of agencies, social connections, cultural ties, and so on that make the picture of an "individual" deciding what to do overly simplistic. Second, I paint a picture of a victimized and vulnerable woman (the formerly trafficked woman) in order to raise issues of paternalism, but in fact many such women have highly developed survival mechanisms, defensive strategies, and other psychological resources at their disposal. Finally, I focus on the paternalistic reasons the aid worker has in trying to decide a course of action, but in most cases such a person will be guided by a complex array of motives and reasons and will be acting within a policy matrix that has its own guidelines and protocols, the prevalence of which may be impossible to sort out precisely in particular cases.

But the fundamental components of the example include the fact that the paternalist is both a potential agent of interference (motivated by concern for the subject) but also is a person who expresses attitudes and provides resources (psychic and otherwise) that are themselves crucial for the subject's capacity to make decisions for herself.

This example is obviously one of asymmetric power. In relations of (more or less) symmetric power, similar dynamics can be in play. As we noted, people in close relations engage in deliberations with a shared intention to allow mutually responsive, norm-guided, reasoning to lead to a decision, without either partner intending a partnership-independent outcome. Insofar as such decisions are central to the life plans of the partners then these sorts of collaborations exercise the autonomy of each and so exhibit the characteristics that give rise to a challenge to the liberal sensibility, namely how respect for autonomy operates when the interaction itself is constitutive of the exercise of that autonomy.

## 5.5 The Challenge for the Liberal Sensibility

The crux of the liberal sensibility I outlined earlier is that the obligation to respect the autonomy of others places limits on the ways that we can intervene into their lives and character development, and that these limits include an attitude of toleration toward the values they (autonomously) embrace. The challenge that asymmetrical partnerships such as that of Seba and Christina pose for this moral sensibility is that while Seba owes Christina respect for the values she might autonomously embrace, a respect that consequently limits the ways she can interact with her, Seba is in the position of shaping the very values and character to which that respect applies.

This challenge, it can be noted, parallels discussions in the realm of liberal education, where a primary directive of facilitating the development of autonomy in children is weighed against (and complicated by) the requirement that education be broadly neutral relative to diverse conceptions of the good life. Harry Brighouse, for example, has argued that education should aim to advance the capacity for autonomy without constraining the person in the development of a wide variety of ways of life (Brighouse 2000). But he claims education should aim to *facilitate* but not *promote* autonomy, since autonomy involves the actual practice of critical self-reflection and such habits may well not be part of a particular person's value structure or orientation. Facilitating autonomy merely helps a person develop the capacities for critical self-reflection but does not induce the actual exercise of those capacities. Indeed, his view has been criticized by those who claim that such capacities cannot be fostered without strongly encouraging actually *using* those abilities; just as one cannot facilitate the disposition for kindness or open-mindedness without inducing people to actually engage in those practices (see, e.g. Corngold 2012).

That worry aside, there is a structural similarity to the tension we are discussing, in that the role of an educator is, arguably, to aid in the development of autonomy related competences and self-defining values, but she or he must also abide by an obligation of tolerance (if not neutrality) toward a wide array of value structures that people might go on to develop by way of that very education. An important contrast, however, is that the vulnerable subjects in partnerships we are imagining are adults (albeit perhaps young adults) with an already established practical identity, fractured though it might be by the trauma and circumstance. Brighouse's directive to facilitate but not promote autonomy may not be effective in cases where aid is required for agents to reassemble a sense of themselves and to establish the capacity to be self-governing in light of this sense.

Recall that the spirit of the liberal sensibility I describe implies that those who are positioned to be instrumental in the development or exercise of the autonomy of another (with whom they are in partnership in my sense) must be guided in that enablement of the others' capacities without expressed judgment of the particular values that might be pursued by that subject. The process of aid whereby the subject regains the capacity for self-government cannot be shaped by an independent appraisal of the quality of the values such self-governing subjects go on to pursue.[14]

This tension arises particularly because the schema for autonomy we are utilizing here attempts to maintain "content neutrality", where the conditions of self-government do not depend on the quality of the values agents are moved by, except insofar as the holding of such values themselves serve to undercut autonomy-related capacities. So appraisal of the inherent quality of the values of the agent themselves is not required to determine her autonomy. But this tension also arises because of the way autonomy has been seen as relational, where interpersonal and social dynamics of particular sorts are claimed to be central to the individual's status as self-governing, as I discussed earlier. As a partner with you, I directly affect the structure and content of the motives that you reflectively accept as your own, and

[14] In other work I looked at this problem specifically with an eye toward the issue of paternalism, asking what limits to paternalism are operative in cases of these sorts of "partnerships". Here I am asking a slightly more general question, namely what is the nature of the obligation to respect others' autonomy, encapsulated in the liberal sensibility, given the ways that one's actions will likely shape the very autonomy which is its object. See Christman 2014a. I also elaborate on partnerships of this sort in Christman 2014b, 231–25.

our relationship may instantiate a dynamic upon which your ability to be autonomous itself depends. Recognition of your status as a self-governing agent able to answer for yourself may in many cases be fundamental in your ability to competently (and confidently) accept her values as her own.

Returning to Bratman's terminology, such shared activity must involve mutual responsiveness, a commitment to the joint activity, and a commitment to mutual support of that activity.[15] The activity I have in mind here is the process of (competent and authentic) deliberation itself. Even in asymmetrical partnerships of the sort I envision, both subjects have the shared intention of helping (at least) one of them develop capabilities and attitudes that allow self-government to be re-established, and hence for the values that she comes to embrace to reflect that self-government.

However, an aid worker such as Seba may well have strong views, for example, on not only the inherent value of practices such as sex work and drug use, but she also must make complex judgments about the relation between being open to going back to such practices and the risk that doing so will undercut Christina's ability to maintain basic competencies of agency that the therapeutic process is designed to re-establish.

Indeed, it has become somewhat of the standard orthodoxy in some therapeutic settings to see the interaction between therapist and client as a dynamic and mutually participatory one. As Stephen Mitchell puts it, the "kind of participation required of the analyst is a complex blend of listening; silently responding; giving oneself over to the explicit and subtle interactional gambits offered by the patient; observing the impact on the patient of one's own ideas and emotional commitments; and giving oneself over to a range of states of mind that allow a broad array of one's own feelings and imaginings" (Mitchell 1997, xii). In this way the therapist is engaged in cooperative deliberation with the patient, one that involves asymmetrical power but which is mutually responsive in Bratman's sense.

The question we must answer, then, is what is the nature and scope of interpersonal respect, called for by the liberal sensibility, in cases of both symmetrical and asymmetrical power when the interpersonal dynamics in question directly affect the establishment or exercise of autonomy?

To answer that question, we should recall that the view of autonomy I described earlier sees that characteristic as not only social but also diachronic, or as described elsewhere "historical." The diachronic view of autonomy sets the conditions of self-government in a way that is sensitive to the ongoing narrative structure of our practical identities. Moreover, autonomy seen in this manner attempts to capture the ways that the authenticity of our current commitments relies importantly on the nature of the processes of value formation that produced them. In short, autonomy amounts to competence (including self-control), and reflectively accepting (without alienation) one's motives in light of their history as part of one's diachronic practical identity.

---

[15] Other accounts that come close to capturing partnerships in my sense include Gilbert 1989 (specifically her account of "plural subjects").

Now even given the complications introduced by the effect that interpersonal power dynamics can have on autonomy, it is easy to see ways in which respect for autonomy can be obviously *violated*. If Seba* (a parallel aid worker), for example, is motivated by a religious conviction that sees prostitution as inherently sinful, so that in addition to helping Christina* regain basic psychological competences and social skills necessary for recovery, she makes it her mission to convince her of that sinfulness, as well as bring her along to the (say) Christian world view that motivates that idea. Such a strategy may well involve imposing a conception of value and the good life that Christina* no longer would share if she were given the chance to competently consider her life options without such pressure.

But if we judge this to be a violation of the respect owed to Christina*, this cannot be based on duties rooted in respect for her *established* autonomous value scheme, for such autonomy is not functioning and its development is dependent on Seba*'s actions themselves. The duty to avoid manipulating vulnerable people to adopt your own world view, then, must be based on respect for what we could call the "nascent autonomy" of the agent. But more to the point, the diachronic, or historical, understanding of autonomy we are using here helps explain this expanded, autonomy-based, duty of respect. The religious devotee that Christina* would become if Seba*'s ministrations were successful would have to accept that position by way of a practical identity that develops over time and embrace that set of (religious) motivations *in light of how they came about*. So only if Christina* would be able to (competently) say that she accepts being a religious person who decries the sinfulness of prostitution, knowing it came about in large part because of the psychological pressures of Seba*'s therapeutic work, would she count as autonomous in the end.

Of course she might so accept such a position: many converts express gratitude toward the influential leaders who brought them to their faith. But only if such reflective acceptance takes place in the full light of the awareness of its origins (among other conditions) is it authentic and so autonomy conferring. In light of such cases, some have criticized the view of autonomy at work here as too permissive, since it seems to allow that a fully manipulated person such as Christina* will count as autonomous as long as the manipulation extends to the acts of historical appraisal itself: any self-respecting manipulator will make sure the person has come to rationalize the process of manipulation itself as part of a grand plan of which she is a part (or some such scenario) (see, e.g., Oshana 2006). But the requirement of eventual self-acceptance in light of one's history I defend is also linked with various other conditions of competence (and competent self-reflection). Such conditions include the ability to consider alternatives, entertain reasons, and avoid overt self-deception. It is unlikely that a person like Christina* will be able to do that without reverting to the self-undercutting rationale of "I did it because that's what I was told".

To elaborate this last point, recall that the model of autonomy I am sketching here demands that the person's eventual reflective self-acceptance must enable her to give reasons that emanate from her diachronic practical identity and which reflexively affirms the values inherent in that identity. That reflective self-acceptance must be in light of the processes (in these cases recovery processes) that allowed her to renegotiate her practical identity. But of course her reflective understanding of herself cannot merely reiterate the psychological results of those processes, so she must be in a position to support her values and commitments independent of them. As I put the point elsewhere, the reflection in question must be sustainable over a variety of conditions and not merely operate because of local and ephemeral causal factors (Christman 2009, 152–3).

So those who are engaged in these sorts of partnership relations are self-governing only if their reflective self-acceptance includes an awareness of those very relations. This is especially true of asymmetrical partnerships. This means that a recovering person like Christina must be able to give, in part at least, *process-independent reasons* in support of the values she comes to hold (and be guided by). To maintain self-government here requires being cognizant of the way that one's development is the result of cooperative reflection and a process of self-constitution with the help of another. The independence from that other – making the resulting self-understanding one's own – requires that one can give reasons for those values independent of the mere fact that one emerged from those therapeutic processes themselves. Only then will the person's reflective self-acceptance meet the adequacy condition mentioned just now, namely that such acceptance is sustainable over a variety of conditions. Being unable to give reasons for one's values independent of the process of forming them ("independent" in the sense of not depending on that process for their justificatory force) would mean that such reflective judgment could not be sustained over a variety of conditions.

This rules out as heteronomous certain sorts of people who emerge from such dependent relations, such as the pure conformist convert who can say nothing in favor of the values she excepts that they accord with what her guru instructed; and at the other end of the spectrum, the recalcitrant rebel who rejects all values as soon as she realizes that some other person influenced her in adopting them.[16] In both cases, the person fails to meet the requirement of reflective self-acceptance here because they cannot give process-independent reasons for holding the views they hold.

Now of course many who go through processes of recovery from trauma may develop emotional dependencies on care-givers and therapists that prevent them from imagining paths other than those that they perceive those therapists would approve of. Perhaps that is the best way to understand what is happening with Christina*. But that, I contend, marks the lack of self-government precisely because she is unable to reflectively answer for herself in ways that both accounts for the process of recovery and is also in some ways independent of it.

Therefore, insofar as the aim of aid workers like Seba should be guided by the (revised) liberal sensibility, then their aim should be that clients and patients come to achieve autonomy in ways that do not manifest the imposition of values that they themselves instigate. That is, they should have as their aim their clients' eventual reflective self-acceptance in light of the process of recovery, reflection whereby the

[16] I am grateful to Ryan Cooke for helping me clarify this point.

clients can give process-independent reasons for their values. In this way, the respect for autonomy underwritten by the liberal sensibility can operate in contexts where interpersonal interaction of this sort has such deep and pervasive effects on the very autonomy being respected.

This conclusion applies to asymmetrical power relationships, but what about other partnerships involving collaborative deliberation that are more or less symmetrical? The claim I made above applies in general form here too, in that the obligation to respect the autonomy of another (with whom one is co-deliberating) amounts to a commitment to a process the end of which would result in a non-alienated narrative self-understanding without reference to the values being pursued by that self. That is, my interaction with my partner involves respectful relations in this sense when I am guided by the norm that says I should make sure our interaction allows her to maintain a sense of herself over time that is undisturbed by an awareness of how our interaction help constitute that sense of self. Diachronic self-acceptance in light of one's history, including a history of interactions that partly constituted the resulting value perspective, is the goal that the obligation to respect the other underwrites.

So those asymmetrical relations where another's autonomy is dependent on one's own actions and attitudes, one has a responsibility to respect the other as a diachronically developing agent, with a past as well as a future, and whose future judgments will be effectively the court of appeal for the respectfulness of one's current interactions. My hope is that such guidelines, even stated in these broad, rough-grained ways, will help reshape duties of respect in all-too-common cases of dependence and vulnerability.

Now it may be thought that a person like Seba giving aid in such situations has just one dominant obligation, namely to advance the well-being of her client, perhaps even including helping her develop autonomy but on the basis of an obligation to *care*, not out of respect for autonomy itself. But this approach fails to capture the obligation to remain respectfully neutral concerning the imposition of particular substantive value schemes expressed in the liberal sensibility. Viewing duties of care-givers as merely the obligation to advance well-being (full stop) would be consistent with such agents' inculcating into their clients a value scheme entirely of their own determination, assuming that it is one that will advance well-being.

More importantly, insofar as the duty to respect autonomy must be refashioned in this way due to the interactive nature of the development and exercise autonomy in such partnerships, the autonomy that is the object of such respect *must* be understood in the diachronic manner I have laid out. Only then can we understand why partners and care-givers have duties to take seriously the autonomous generation of values and choices of the other even when their activity dynamically constitutes that autonomy. If we viewed autonomy as a time-slice characteristic, or as a trait impervious to the processes of its development, then the obligation to respect others as autonomous would gain no foothold in the partnership interactions we have envisioned, and Seba* would have done no wrong to Christina*. But surely she does.

What I have argued here, then, is that in partnerships of the sort I have described, the duties associated with the liberal sensibility – to respect autonomy of others – must be complicated by a provision taking account of the ways that interpersonal and social interaction are themselves constituents of autonomy. Hence, our obligations to respect the autonomy of others when we have power over their development of that very autonomy must take on a diachronic mode, namely that we must aim to facilitate the development of a practical identity which can be the basis of future judgments that would not be disturbed when considered in light of that very process of interaction and facilitation.

Autonomy is a cooperative enterprise in many ways, and only if we engage in this enterprise in caring and respectful ways, sensitive to the complex manner in which social interactions shape the very persons we are, will self-government emerge as the morally noteworthy capacity it is thought to be.[17]

## References

Anderson, Joel, and Axel Honneth. 2005. Autonomy, Vulnerability, Recognition, and Justice. In *Autonomy and the Challenges to Liberalism: New Essays*, ed. John Christman and Joel Anderson, 127–149. Cambridge: Cambridge University Press.

Benson, Paul. 2005. Taking Ownership: Authority and Voice in Autonomous Agency. In *Autonomy and the Challenges to Liberalism: New Essays*, ed. John Christman and Joel Anderson, 101–126. Cambridge: Cambridge University Press.

Bratman, Michael. 2007. *Structures of Agency*. Oxford: Oxford University Press.

———. 2014. *Shared Agency: A Planning Theory of Acting Together*. Oxford: Oxford University Press.

Brighouse, Harry. 2000. *School Choice and Social Justice*. Oxford: Oxford University Press.

Brison, Susan. 2003. *Aftermath: Violence and the Remaking of Ourselves*. Princeton, NJ: Princeton University Press.

Christman, John. 2009. *The Politics of Persons: Individual Autonomy and Socio-historical Selves*. Cambridge: Cambridge University Press.

———. 2014a. Relational Autonomy and the Social Dynamics of Paternalism. *Ethical Theory and Moral Practice* 17: 3690–3682. (special issue edited by Annete Dufner and Michael Kuhler).

———. 2014b. Freedom and the Extended Self. *Ethical Perspectives* 21 (2): 225–254.

Christman, John, and Joel Anderson, eds. 2005. *Autonomy and the Challenges to Liberalism: New Essays*. Cambridge: Cambridge University Press.

Corngold, Josh. 2012. Autonomy-facilitation or Autonomy-promotion? The case of Sex Education. *Theory and Research in Education* 10 (1(March)): 157–170.

Dworkin, Gerald. 1989. *The Theory and Practice of Autonomy*. Cambridge: Cambridge University Press.

Frankfurt, Harry. 1987. Freedom of the Will and the Concept of a Person. In *The Importance of What We Care About*. Cambridge: Cambridge University Press.

———. 1992. The Faintest Passion. *Proceedings and Addresses of the Aristotelian Society* 49: 113–145.

———. 1999. *Necessity, Volition, and Love*. Cambridge: Cambridge University Press.

Gilbert, Margaret. 1989. *On Social Facts*. Princeton: Princeton University Press.

[17] This paper is a revised version of a paper given at the conference: Thick Concepts of Autonomy. Center for Advanced Study in Bioethics. University of Muenster, Germany. October 18–20, 2012. I am grateful to Michael Quante, Thomas Gutmann, Johann Ach, and Bettina Schoene-Seifert for organizing the conference and to all participants for very helpful discussion and commentary.

Kristinsson, S. 2000. The Limits of Neutrality: Toward a Weakly Substantive Account of Autonomy. *Canadian Journal of Philosophy* 30 (2) (June): 257–286.
Korsgaard, Christine 1996. *The Sources of Normativity*. Cambridge: Cambridge University Press.
Lear, Jonathan. 2006. *Radical Hope: Ethics in the Face of Cultural Devastation*. Cambridge, MA: Harvard University Press.
Mackenzie, Catriona. 2008. Relational Autonomy, Normative Authority and Perfectionism. *Journal of Social Philosophy* 39: 512–533.
Mele, Al. 1995. *Autonomous Agents: From Self-Control to Autonomy*. New York: Oxford University Press.
Mitchell, Stephen. 1997. *Influence and Autonomy in Psychoanalysis*. London: Routledge.
Oshana, Marina. 2006. *Personal Autonomy in Society*. Hampshire: Ashgate Publishing.
Sandel, Michael. 1982. *Liberalism and the Limits of Justice*. Cambridge: Cambridge University Press.
Westlund, Andrea. 2003. Selflessness and Responsibility for Self: Is Deference Compatible with Autonomy? *The Philosophical Review* 112 (4(October)): 483–523.

Mulhall, Stephen. 1996. *Heidegger and Being and Time*. London: Routledge.

# Chapter 6
# Autonomy and Beliefs

**Alfred R. Mele**

**Abstract** In *Autonomous Agents*, I argued that among the obstacles to autonomous action are facts of certain kinds about an agent's beliefs. For example, someone who is deceived into investing her savings in a way that results in her losing the entire investment to the person who deceived her may correctly be said to make that investment nonautonomously. But not everyone has agreed. In this article, I return to doxastic aspects of individual autonomy and argue more fully for the thesis that facts of a certain kind about an agent's beliefs can render some of an agent's actions nonautonomous.

King George just now issued a decree raising property taxes by five percent throughout his kingdom. What would suffice for his doing that autonomously? And what would suffice for his doing that nonautonomously? In *Autonomous Agents* (Mele 1995, pp. 180–82), I suggested that certain facts about George's beliefs might render the specified action nonautonomous. My view about this has been challenged (McKenna 2005, Weimer 2009), and I return to doxastic aspects of individual autonomy in this article.

Before I get down to business, I should point out that philosophers use the term "autonomy" in a variety of senses, even when only autonomous individuals (rather than nations, for example) are at issue.[1] The root idea of autonomy – from *autos* (self) and *nomos* (rule or law) – is self-rule or self-government. My attempt to understand autonomous action in Mele 1995 is primarily an attempt to understand the nature of actions distinctive of self-ruled or self-governed individuals. "Autonomy," as I use

[1] Joel Feinberg usefully distinguishes among four "meanings" of "autonomy" as applied to individuals (1986, p. 28). Also see Arpaly 2003, pp. 118–2.

A. R. Mele (✉)
Department of Philosophy, Florida State University, Tallahassee, FL, USA
e-mail: amele@fsu.edu



J. F. Childress, M. Quante (eds.), *Thick (Concepts of) Autonomy*, Philosophical Studies Series 146, https://doi.org/10.1007/978-3-030-80991-1_6

the term there (as applied to individuals) is in the family of metaphysical freedom terms: "free will," "free choice," "free action," and the like. I use it the same way here.

## 6.1 Autonomous and Nonautonomous Actions: Setting Things Up

Some background information about King George is in order (see Mele 1995, p. 180). Through no fault of his own, the only access George has to his kingdom is through his staff of advisors. His primary concern in life is to do what is best for his kingdom as a whole. The staff provide him with information, and he takes legislative and other measures on that basis. They also provide George with feedback about his measures, which information he takes into account in drafting further legislation and in modifying previous measures. They give him monthly figures on a variety of matters, including the gross national product, the distribution of wealth, the percentage of the population living below the poverty level, the King's popularity, and the popular reaction to his legislative acts. However the staff have their own agenda – namely, their own enrichment at the expense of the populace. Knowing the King's preferences, they systematically provide him with false information that will lead him to make decisions that will further their aims. Of course, they are careful not to be so obvious about this as to call their loyalty into question.

Today, George's advisors presented him with information they knew would lead him to conclude that his issuing a decree raising property taxes by five percent would put an end to poverty in his kingdom while not greatly inconveniencing anyone. George rationally drew that conclusion, and he issued such a decree. The advisors kept the new tax revenues for themselves, as they planned all along to do; and they knew that even if the proceeds had gone to the poor, poverty would have continued to be a serious problem in the kingdom. Most landowners are in debt to wage earners – especially to the King's advisors. A raise in income taxes (rather than property taxes) would have helped significantly with poverty in the kingdom (provided the money actually went to the poor). In their subsequent monthly reports to George, his advisors provide very encouraging news about shrinking poverty figures.

In my view, issuing the tax decree is not something George autonomously does. By controlling what George believes about the effect a five percent raise in property taxes will have, his staff gain control over whether he will judge it best to issue the decree and whether he will issue it (see Mele 1995, pp. 180–82). In light of the control his advisors exert here, I see George as heteronomous in this connection.

Am I wrong about this? Michael McKenna spins a story that is intended to shed light on George's situation. In it, Tal tries to save Daphne's life by giving her "the prescribed dose" from "a bottle marked 'The Good Stuff'" (2005, p. 209). Tal has every reason to believe that the medication will help Daphne and no reason to believe that it will harm her. Unfortunately, the bottle is accidentally mislabeled. It contains a drug that is lethal for a person with Daphne's illness: Tal kills Daphne by giving her the drug. McKenna reports that this story "helps to confirm the need for [an] epistemic condition on morally responsible agency" (p. 209). He also asks whether "Tal acted nonautonomously in giving Daphne the drug" (p. 210). The answer he seems to endorse is no: he acted autonomously "in giving Daphne the drug" (pp. 210–11).

Consider the following true sentences:

Tal gave Daphne the prescribed dose from a bottle marked "The Good Stuff"
Tal gave Daphne a lethal (for her) drug
Tal killed Daphne

Insert "autonomously" immediately after "Tal" in each sentence. Which (if any) of the resulting sentences are true? Some readers may experience some uncertainty about how to answer. A brief review of a basic issue in the philosophy of action may help.

Donald Davidson writes: "I flip the switch, turn on the light, and illuminate the room. Unbeknownst to me I also alert a prowler to the fact that I am home" (1980, p. 4). How many actions has the agent, Don, performed? Davidson's *coarse-grained* answer is one action "of which four descriptions have been given" (p. 4). A *fine-grained* alternative treats *A* and *B* as different actions if, in performing them, the agent exemplifies different act-properties (Goldman 1970). On this view, Don performs at least four actions, since the act-properties at issue are distinct. For example, the property of flipping a switch is distinct from the property of turning on a light, and the property of turning on a light (in a room) is distinct from the property of illuminating a room. One may flip a switch without turning on a light and vice versa. Similarly, one may turn on a light in a room without illuminating the room (the light may be painted black) and illuminate a room without turning on a light (by setting a dark room on fire). Another alternative – a componential one – represents Don's illuminating the room as an action having various components, including (but not limited to) his moving his arm (an action), his flipping the switch (an action), and the light's going on (Ginet 1990; Thalberg 1977; Thomson 1977). Where proponents of the coarse-grained and fine-grained theories find, respectively, a single action under different descriptions and a collection of intimately related actions, advocates of the various componential views locate a "larger" action having "smaller" actions among its parts.

When actions are individuated in Davidson's coarse-grained way, it is *actions under descriptions* that are performed intentionally or otherwise – not actions period. Similarly, it is actions under descriptions that are performed for a reason *R* (or for a reason at all). For example, under the description "flips the switch," what Don does is intentional; but under the description "alerts the prowler," what he does is not intentional. Similarly, under the description "flips the switch," Don might have acted for a reason having to do with getting sufficient light to find his keys; but under the description "alerts the prowler," Don does not act for a reason at all (Davidson 1980, p. 5).

Fine-grained and componential theorists make no special appeal to action-descriptions. Theorists of both kinds can straightforwardly say, for example, that Don intentionally flipped the switch, unintentionally alerted the prowler, and flipped the switch in order to have enough light to find his keys and that, although he alerted the prowler, he did not do that for a reason.

Might "autonomously" work in a way that resembles the way in which "intentionally" and "for a reason" work? Might it be the case, for example, that although Don autonomously flips the switch, autonomously turns on the light, autonomously illuminates the room, and alerts the prowler (by illuminating the room), he does not autonomously alert the prowler? Framed in Davidsonian terms, might it be the case that what Don does is autonomously done under the descriptions "flips the switch," "turns on the light," and "illuminates the room" but not under the description "alerts the prowler"?

An easy way to avoid saying a lot of things twice – both in terms of Davidson's coarse-grained theory of action individuation and in non-Davidsonian terms – is to invite readers to understand the action variable "*A*" as a variable for actions themselves (construed componentially or otherwise) or actions under descriptions, depending on their preferred theory of action individuation. The same goes for the expressions that take the place of "*A*" in concrete examples. For example, proponents of Davidson's theory should read "Don illuminates the room" as "something Don does under the description 'illuminates the room'" and non-Davidsonians should make no adjustments. I proceed on the assumption that readers accept my invitation. Readers who have no preferred theory of action individuation should feel free to adopt one temporarily.

McKenna asks (2005, p. 210): "Should we reconsider the case of Tal and, consistent with Mele's intuitions about … King George, conclude that Tal acted nonautonomously in giving Daphne the drug?" His answer is no. But it is difficult to be sure exactly what McKenna has in mind by the expression "in giving Daphne the drug." Suppose we change "in" to "when" in the clause just quoted. We might then say that Tal did some things autonomously and some other things nonautonomously at that time. In the former group, some might confidently place his giving Daphne the prescribed dose from a bottle marked "The Good Stuff." In the latter, I would confidently place his giving Daphne a lethal (for her) drug, and his killing Daphne.

It might have occurred to some readers that if the three placements in the preceding paragraph are correct, what is doing the work is the difference between intentional and nonintentional action. It is true that Tal intentionally gives Daphne the prescribed dose from a bottle marked "The Good Stuff" and that he neither intentionally gives her a lethal (for her) drug nor intentionally kills her. Even so, the claim about what is doing the work is open to criticism.

Consider the following case:

> Unbeknownst to Bob, who intends to vote Democratic, the Democratic lever in his voting booth is attached to a randomizing device. The only way for him to vote Democratic is to pull that lever, but pulling the lever yields only a 0.001 chance of producing a Democratic vote. Luckily, Bob succeeds in registering a vote for the Democratic candidate. (Mele 1995, p. 14, n. 11)

As I see it, Bob's producing that vote was too lucky to count as an intentional action, even though that is what he intended to do (see Mele and Moser 1994). Even so, if Bob autonomously decided to vote for the Democrat and autonomously pulled the lever, I see no compelling reason to deny that he *autonomously* (or freely) produced a Democratic vote.

That is why I would not infer merely from its being true that Tal did not intentionally kill Daphne that he did not kill her autonomously. But, of course, there is an important difference between the stories about Bob and Tal in this connection. Bob intended – and was trying – to register a vote for the Democrat, and Tal neither intended nor tried to kill Daphne. As far as I can see, the judgment that Tal did not autonomously kill Daphne is extremely plausible, as is the judgment that he did not autonomously give her a lethal (for her) drug.

Return to George. The following sentences are true of him:

George raised property taxes by five percent
George enriched his advisors

Insert "autonomously" immediately after "George" in both sentences. Which (if any) of the resulting sentences are true?

The judgment that George did not autonomously enrich his advisors (by raising taxes) is at least as plausible as the judgment that Tal did not autonomously kill Daphne. George neither intended nor tried to enrich his advisors (by raising taxes). He unintentionally enriched them. And, of course, he was tricked into enriching them.

Did George autonomously raise taxes by five percent? Earlier in this section I denied that he did on grounds having to do with the control his advisors exerted over him. McKenna contends that if "we are interested in action-theoretic questions about whether certain sorts of persons have the capacity to guide their own conduct in light of rules that they themselves endorse, it is hard to see how the sorts of epistemic pollutants presented to King George could foul up [his] having acted in such a manner" (2005, p. 228, n. 13). Let us stipulate that George has the capacity McKenna mentions and that he often guides his behavior in a variety of spheres in light of rules he endorses. It is hard to see how this fact about George undermines the claim that he did not autonomously raise taxes. Presumably, this fact about George is no obstacle at all to the claim that he nonautonomously enriched his advisors. This is so even if, at the pertinent time, George was exercising a "capacity to guide [his] own conduct in light of rules" he endorsed – perhaps, in this instance, a rule favoring trying to help the poor in his kingdom. So, why, exactly, should the fact at issue be thought to undermine the claim that George nonautonomously raised property taxes? Does the answer feature the fact that George intentionally raised property taxes? The action-theoretic questions that interest me at present are about the status of particular actions: for example, the question whether George autonomously raised taxes.

In a passage to which the note from which I just quoted is appended, McKenna identifies agents' "ruling themselves in acting as they do" with their acting "in light of rules that they themselves accept as their own" (2005, pp. 210–11). Now, at a time at which one is acting in light of a rule that one endorses (that is, accepts as one's own), one may be doing some things intentionally and other things unintentionally. For example, Don endorses a rule in favor of always turning on a light when he enters his kitchen. Just now, he acted in light of that rule. He flipped a switch in his kitchen and turned on a light. Unfortunately, an enemy who knew Don's habits wired the switch to a bomb he placed in Don's oven. When Don flipped the switch, he detonated the bomb and blew up his house. Although he flipped the switch and turned on the light intentionally, he detonated the bomb and blew up his house unintentionally. And, again, it may be that just as one can do some things intentionally while doing other things unintentionally, one can do some things autonomously while doing other things nonautonomously.

McKenna supposes, to keep things simple, that when Tal gave Daphne the lethal drug, he was "consciously acting" from the following "principle that he endorsed": "Always attempt to help those who are suffering innocently" (2005, p. 209). At that time, then, in McKenna's view, Tal was acting in light of a rule that he accepts as his own and ruling himself in acting as he did. Even if this were to suffice for Tal's autonomously doing something or other at the time – perhaps, attempting to save Daphne's life – that would leave it open that Tal nonautonomously does various other things at the same time. My concern, again, is with what is and is not done autonomously at a time – not simply with whether an agent is doing something or other autonomously at a time.

McKenna contends that "*if* there is an epistemic constraint on autonomous agency, it differs from the sort of epistemic constraint pertinent to morally responsible agency" (2005, p. 211). "It is reasonable to assume," he writes, "that morally responsible agency requires two sorts of conditions: an epistemic and a control condition" (p. 207). He understands the latter condition "in terms of the freedom of the will" (p. 208), and he tells us that "freely willed action" does not "involve a significant epistemic component" (p. 211).[2] McKenna writes: "Perhaps careful investigation will reveal that self-ruling agency just is, or is a component of, freely willing agency. If so, it would be correct to conclude that autonomous action does not involve a significant epistemic component because freely willed action does not" (p. 211).

In a note to the sentence I quoted about the assumption that "morally responsible agency requires an epistemic and a control condition," McKenna (2005, p. 228, n. 7) cites "Aristotle's conditions on the voluntary from *Nicomachean Ethics* … 1109b30–1111b5" and a related discussion in Fischer and Ravizza 1998 (pp. 12–14). Attention to a pair of ironies about these citations will prove instructive.

Aristotle (1915) writes: "Since that which is done under compulsion or by reason of ignorance is involuntary, the voluntary would seem to be that of which the moving principle is in the agent himself, he being aware of the particular circumstances of the action" (*Nicomachean Ethics* 1111a22–24). Now, in ordinary English, what

[2] McKenna backs away from this claim about free (or "freely willed") action in his recent book (2012, p. 13).

is said to be done voluntarily seems to be more tightly connected to what is said to be done freely or autonomously than to what people are said to be morally responsible for doing. In an ordinary drunk driver scenario in which the driver is too drunk even to see the pedestrian he runs down, it is generally claimed that the driver is morally responsible for running down the pedestrian even though he did not voluntarily run the unfortunate person down. But the suggestion that a person does something autonomously (or freely) only if he does it voluntarily has a very plausible ring. Accordingly, Aristotle's view about the voluntary seems congruent with the claim that there are significant epistemic requirements for autonomous actions and free actions.

The second irony concerns the discussion by John Fischer and Mark Ravizza that McKenna cites and related work by Fischer (alone or with a coauthor). Fischer and Ravizza report that "the focus of … attention" in their book is "the freedom-relevant condition on moral responsibility, rather than the epistemic condition" (1998, p. 13; also see Fischer 1994, p. 238, n. 4). The epistemic condition "corresponds to the excuse of ignorance. It captures the intuition that an agent is responsible only if he both knows the particular facts surrounding his action, and acts with the proper sorts of beliefs and intentions" (p. 13). "The freedom-relevant condition specifies that the agent must control his behavior in a suitable sense, in order to be morally responsible for it" (p. 13).

As I have explained elsewhere (Mele 2010), Fischer and his coauthors have not specified epistemic requirements for being morally responsible for *A*-ing that they clearly regard as not also being requirements for freely *A*-ing. Furthermore, their "freedom-relevant condition" – or "control condition" (Fischer and Ravizza 1998, p. 13) – has some notable epistemic features, including the agent's having at least one mechanism that can recognize moral reasons and the agent's not being substantially deluded about the nature of reality (see Mele 2010). Even if, in McKenna's words, "morally responsible agency requires an epistemic and a control condition" (2005, p. 207), work by Fischer and coauthors thus far seems to leave it open that any necessary epistemic conditions for an agent's being morally responsible for *A*-ing are also necessary conditions for the agent's freely – or autonomously – *A*-ing.[3] This is the second irony to which I referred.

A related observation is in order. Compare a kleptomaniac, Karen, who has, through no fault of her own, an irresistible desire to steal a necklace with a man, Dan, who is nonculpably ignorant of a certain important fact – that a party he has been invited to is a surprise party (see Fischer and Tognazzini 2009, p. 531–32 and Mele 2010, pp. 109–10). The former steals the necklace and the latter spoils the surprise by talking about the upcoming party to the person who was meant to be surprised. Karen is not blameworthy for stealing the necklace, and Dan is not blameworthy for ruining the surprise. The excuses are of two very different kinds. Karen's excuse is that she was forced to steal by an irresistible desire and therefore did not

[3] I am not denying that there are necessary epistemic conditions for being a morally responsible agent that are not necessary conditions for being a free agent. For discussion, see Mele 2010, pp. 108–9.

freely steal; and what excuses Dan for spoiling the party was nonculpable ignorance of a crucial fact. Dan's excuse is epistemic and Karen's is not. But it should not be inferred from this that Dan freely ruined the surprise – that his ruining the surprise was a free action.[4] Just as Karen's being compelled to steal makes it true that she did not freely steal, Dan's ignorance might make it true that he did not freely ruin the surprise. The fact that there are legitimate "control"-based excuses and very different "ignorance"-based excuses does not itself straightforwardly entail that there are epistemic requirements for being morally responsible for *A*-ing that are not also requirements for freely – or autonomously – *A*-ing.

## 6.2 Sorting Through Cases

Return to McKenna's claim that Tal acted autonomously "in giving Daphne the drug" (2005, pp. 210–11). Suppose the bottle that was accidentally marked "The Good Stuff" contained labeled pills. Tal found three pills in the bottle – labeled GS8, GS9, and GS10. He decided to give Daphne what he assumed was the next pill in the sequence of pills she had been taking – GS8. One can ask whether Tal acted autonomously "in giving Daphne" GS8, as McKenna might. Or one can ask simply whether he autonomously gave her GS8. I choose the latter question. Whether a *yes* answer to this question is true or false, it at least does not *sound* terribly implausible. It does not sound as implausible as, for example, a *yes* answer to the question whether Tal autonomously killed Daphne.

Consider a modified version of Tal's story. Daphne's mother, Molly, is in the room when Daphne has a seizure. Molly is confined to a wheelchair and moves too slowly to help Daphne. Tal asks Molly what he should do. She tells him to get pill GS8 from the bottle on Daphne's dresser and give it to her. Tal has every reason to believe that Molly wants to save Daphne; but, in fact, she wants her dead. Molly knows that GS8 is lethal for anyone in Daphne's condition. Tal gives Daphne GS8, thereby killing her.

Did Tal autonomously give Daphne GS8 in this modified story? Was his giving her that pill an autonomous action? I say *no*. To be heteronomous regarding something is to be ruled or dominated by another agent (or other agents) regarding it. Molly is in control of how Tal seeks to solve Daphne's urgent problem; and I see him, accordingly, as heteronomously giving Daphne GS8. He has become Molly's

[4] Readers will, of course, distinguish Dan's saying what he does about the party from his ruining the surprise. For example, they will notice that even if it is assumed that he intentionally says what he does about the party, he does not intentionally ruin the surprise. Incidentally, in the paragraph that precedes Aristotle's assertion that "the voluntary would seem to be that of which the moving principle is in the agent himself, he being aware of the particular circumstances of the action" (*Nicomachean Ethics* 1111a22–24), he mentions an agent who "did not know" that what he reported "was a secret" (1111a9–10). I take it that he would say that, owing to his ignorance of this circumstance, this agent did not voluntarily reveal a secret. If it is true that he did not voluntarily reveal a secret, then if we freely do only what we voluntarily do, he did not freely reveal a secret.

tool for killing Daphne. If Tal heteronomously gives Daphne GS8, he does not do it autonomously (which is not to say, of course, that he does not do anything autonomously at the time).

There is no obvious contradiction in claiming that Tal autonomously gives Daphne GS8 in McKenna's story but not in mine. But is there a troubling tension? In my discussion of a radical kind of manipulation in Mele 1995 – a kind in which manipulators intentionally erase a person's core values and replace them with radically different values (with a certain property that need not concern the reader now) – I say that the resulting nonautonomy (regarding various actions) would also result if the same transformation in a person's values were produced by blind forces: for example, a bizarre electromagnetic storm (pp. 168–69). Steven Weimer contends that I should take a similar approach on the informational front (2009, pp. 29–30). In his view, I should avoid endorsing a view according to which the difference between whether someone did something autonomously or nonautonomously sometimes depends on whether important false beliefs of his are or are not products of intentional deception.[5] So, for example, if I say that in McKenna's story about Tal, where there is no intentional deception, Tal autonomously gives Daphne GS8, I should say the same in my story.

Suppose I were to say that I am agnostic about whether Tal autonomously gives Daphne GS8 in McKenna's story. Would that put enormous pressure on me to say – symmetrically – that I am agnostic about whether Tal autonomously gives Daphne GS8 in my story?

An attempt to answer this question may benefit from attention to some "bad information" scenarios that have a feature in common with the manipulation stories of mine to which Weimer refers and with counterpart stories featuring blind forces. Recall that in the pertinent stories, the agents' core values are erased and replaced by very different values. One might do well to consider stories in which crucial beliefs are erased and replaced by very different beliefs.

Here is a third version of Tal's story. In this version, Tal had learned that when Daphne has a seizure, he needs to give her a pill is the *S* series. What he learned is true; but, as part of her plan for bringing about Daphne's death, Molly hired someone to knock out Tal's true belief about this and replace it with the belief that the correct pill for seizures is any pill in the *GS* series.[6] She then induced a seizure in Daphne. Tal gave Daphne GS8, thereby killing her. In this case, in my opinion, Tal is heteronomous with respect to his giving Daphne GS8 and therefore gives it to her nonautonomously. Here, as in my earlier story about him, Tal has become Molly's tool for killing Daphne.

In a fourth version of Tal's story, a bizarre electromagnetic storm does the belief-replacing work. Molly induces a seizure in Daphne, believing that Tal will not be there to try to save her; but Tal shows up in time to act on his new belief. Tal is not

[5] Suzy Killmister takes the approach Weimer recommends on the informational front (2013, p. 517 n. 4).

[6] On some complications about belief replacement, see Mele 2006, pp. 177–78.

heteronomous with respect to his giving Daphne GS8: no other agent has taken control of what he does. That leaves it open that giving Daphne GS8 is not something he autonomously does. But it also leaves it open that he autonomously gives her GS8.

Suppose for the sake of argument that Tal autonomously gives Daphne GS8 in the version of the story in which the bottle of pills is accidentally mislabeled and the version featuring the strange storm. Is the truth of that supposition compatible with it also being true that Tal nonautonomously gives her GS8 in the other two versions of the story (the version in which Molly lies and the version in which Tal's true belief about the needed medication is intentionally knocked out and replaced by a false belief)? At first sight, at least, the answer to this question about compatibility would seem to be *yes*. There is a salient difference between the two pairs of stories: in one pair Tal, has been intentionally manipulated (by means of intentional deception or intentional belief replacement); and in the other pair, this is not the case. That difference may help to explain how Tal can autonomously give Daphne GS8 in two of the stories but not in the other two.

This brings us back to the idea that just as I make symmetrical judgments about certain value-manipulation stories and comparable value-change stories featuring "blind forces," I should make symmetrical judgments about the four stories about Tal. Is this correct? To pursue this question, I need to say something about how I understand values and tell a story about value manipulation.

As I understand valuing, "*S* at least *thinly values X* at a time if and only if at that time *S* both has a positive motivational attitude toward *X* and believes *X* to be good" (Mele 1995, p. 116). When values are understood as psychological states, I take them to have both of these dimensions by definition. This account of thinly valuing and the corresponding thin account of values are not intended as contributions to the theories of valuing and values; their purpose is to make my meaning clear.

The following story about value manipulation will do. I call it "One Good Day" (see Mele 2009, p. 471; for a similar story, see Mele 1995, pp. 164–65).

Chuck enjoys killing people, and he "is wholeheartedly behind" his murderous desires, which are "well integrated into his general psychic condition" (Frankfurt 2002, p. 27). When he kills, he does so "because he wants to do it" (Frankfurt 2002, p. 27), and "he identifies himself with the springs of his action" (Frankfurt 1988, p. 54). When he was much younger, Chuck enjoyed torturing animals, but he was not wholeheartedly behind this. These activities sometimes caused him to feel guilty, he experienced bouts of squeamishness, and he occasionally considered abandoning animal torture. However, Chuck valued being the sort of person who does as he pleases and who unambivalently rejects conventional morality as a system designed for and by weaklings. He freely set out to ensure that he would be wholeheartedly behind his torturing of animals and related activities, including his merciless bullying of vulnerable people, and he was morally responsible for so doing. One strand of his strategy was to perform cruel actions with increased frequency in order to harden himself against feelings of guilt and squeamishness and eventually to extinguish the source of those feelings. Chuck strove to ensure that his psyche left no room for mercy. His strategy worked. In hardening his heart as he did,

Chuck also ensured that he had no values at all that could motivate a charitable deed. (He might buy some Girl Scout cookies to lure an innocent child away for evil purposes; but a cookie-buying motivated in that way is not a charitable deed.)

A high-powered team of scientists captured Chuck and ran an experiment on him. They had identified the system of values of an extremely sweet and generous woman, Beth; and they wanted to learn whether they could erase Chuck's nasty values and replace them with values like Beth's. The plan was to do this while Chuck slept, turn him loose for a day, and then restore his old values at midnight. Things worked perfectly. Shortly after he awoke, Chuck started working with a local Habitat for Humanity crew in his neighborhood. He worked long and hard, feeling very good about what he was doing. When the work day ended, he drove around town for an hour and bought several boxes of Girl Scout cookies from every Girl Scout he saw – about fifty boxes in all. Then he delivered the cookies to a local homeless shelter. His motives were pure, as Beth's are when she does her charitable deeds. Naturally, Chuck wondered about the remarkable change in himself. His explanation was that he had finally seen the light about how to live. Occasionally, he reflected on his new values and wholeheartedly endorsed them. The scientists predicted the endorsement. After all, any process of critical reflection is conducted from some perspective or other; and Chuck's wonderful new values dominate the perspective from which reflects on his values in such a way that continued identification with them is ensured.

Does Chuck autonomously work with Habitat for Humanity, help Girl Scouts, and feed the homeless on his one good day? The intuitive answer is *no*, or so it seems to me. Presumably, if it is true that Chuck autonomously performs the charitable actions at issue, then he deserves some moral credit for those actions, as Beth does for hers. Does he deserve credit for them? Knowing what you do about the source of those actions, would you give him moral credit for performing them? I doubt it – unless, perhaps, you endorse a theory that commits you to doing so. And why would you not give him such credit? Because he does not deserve it, it seems.

Consider now a variant of One Good Day in which a strange electromagnetic storm (or a weird cluster of brain tumors) has the effect on Chuck's values that the scientists achieved in the original story. Chuck does everything he does in the first story – including reflectively endorsing his new values – and he feels the same way about his activities. At the end of the day, all of the changes in his values are undone. Chuck is back to normal – for him, that is.

Here too, it seems, Chuck deserves no moral credit for his good deeds. They are the product of values that swept into him over night and that he had no role at all in producing or shaping.[7] Moreover, the values that guide his behavior on his one good day are utterly contrary to values that he did play a part in shaping – the core values of his that were erased by the strange storm. Now, presumably, if it were true that Chuck performs his charitable actions autonomously, he would deserve some moral

[7] I am not claiming that one has to be responsible for attitudes if one is to be responsible for behavior in which the attitudes issue. On this topic, see Mele 1995, pp. 221–230.

credit for them (as Beth does for hers). From his deserving no such credit for them, we can infer that he does not autonomously perform them.

In my first story about Chuck, the claim that he is heteronomous with respect to his good behavior is plausible. There, the scientists seize control of (some of) what he does by instilling wonderful Beth-like values in him. In my second story about Chuck, no other agents seize control. The drastic, temporary change in his value system is a product of blind forces. He does not heteronomously perform his charitable deeds; but he does not autonomously perform them either, if I am right.

*If* it is correct to judge that Chuck's good deeds are nonautonomously performed in both stories about him but incorrect to make symmetrical judgments about Tal's giving Daphne GS8 in the four stories about him, why might that be? In the absence of a reasonable answer, those who have symmetrical intuitions about Chuck but asymmetrical intuitions about Tal should worry that some of these intuitions are misguided.

Where there are differences in responses to stories (even if the difference is between agnostic and non-agnostic responses), we should look for differences in the stories that might reasonably account for them. In the pair of stories about Chuck, his entire moral personality, as it were, has been radically reversed – either intentionally or accidentally. In the quartet of stories about Tal, the featured psychological matter is very localized, and it is in a different sphere – the sphere of beliefs about relatively simple matters of fact. These differences between the Chuck stories and the Tal stories are obvious ones, but do these differences have a significant bearing on autonomous action?

Suppose that value reversal of the kind and magnitude present in Chuck's stories precludes his autonomously performing his good deeds. It certainly does not follow from the truth of this supposition that, for example, the changes in belief in my last two stories about Tal preclude his autonomously giving Daphne GS8. The two kinds of change – that is, radical change in moral personality and change in a belief about pills – are so different that the inference at issue is, at best, far-fetched. Now, it is a truism that if one is heteronomous with respect to one's *A*-ing, one does not autonomously *A*. A reader who sees Tal as heteronomous with respect to his giving Daphne GS8 in the story in which his relevant true belief is intentionally knocked out and replaced with a belief that the correct pill for Daphne's seizures is any pill in the *GS* series and in the story in which Molly deceives him into believing that GS8 will save her will deny that he autonomously gives Daphne GS8 in these stories. But when that reader turns to the other two stories about Tal, in which he is not heteronomous, this particular route to the claim that Tal nonautonomously gives Daphne GS8 is closed, and the reader is faced with a difficult question, a question related to one raised by a remark by Aristotle that I quoted earlier: "the voluntary would seem to be that of which the moving principle is in the agent himself, he being aware of the particular circumstances of the action" (*Nicomachean Ethics* 1111a22–24).

Circumstances of what kind? Aristotle says a bit about this, and one of his illustrations is especially fitting in the present context: "one might give a man a draught to save him, and really kill him" (1111a 13–14). But is he claiming merely that agent does not voluntarily kill the man or also that he does not voluntarily give the man the drink he gives him – does not voluntarily *give the man D*, for short? And, whatever Aristotle might have thought about this, what should we think? Again, it is plausible that one *A*-s autonomously only if one *A*-s voluntarily. So a reader who is unsure whether to accept or reject the claim that this agent voluntarily gives the man D may also be uncertain about whether he does this autonomously. And the very same reader may be confident that in a version of Aristotle's story in which, in order to bring about the man's death, someone deceived the agent into believing that the lethal liquid would save the man, the agent does not autonomously give the man D.

I plead ignorance about whether, in the non-heteronomy stories, the agent just discussed voluntarily gives the man D and Tal voluntarily gives Daphne GS8. But my being ignorant about this does not entail that I am mistaken in holding that, in the versions of these stories that feature deception or intentional belief replacement, the agent nonautonomously gives the man D and Tal nonautonomously gives Daphne GS8.

What brought me to this point was an investigation prompted by Weimer's contention that just as I take a symmetrical position regarding autonomous action in value-change stories like my two stories about Chuck (one of which features intentionally induced value change whereas the other features a matching change in values induced by blind forces), I should do the same in the informational sphere. I have tried to motivate a rejection of this contention. My own grip on a notion of autonomous action leaves me agnostic about whether Tal autonomously gives Daphne GS8 in the non-heteronomy stories even though I claim that he nonautonomously does this in the other stories. This is an asymmetrical position, and I have argued that it is compatible with my symmetrical position on the Chuck stories.

I started with King George. What does this have to do with him? In my view (see Mele 1995, pp. 180–82), he does not autonomously issue the decree raising property taxes by five percent. McKenna, partly by means of his discussion of his story about Tal, argues that this view of mine is mistaken (2005). Here, I have explained why McKenna's argument is unpersuasive even if it is granted that Tal autonomously gives Daphne GS8 in a story like his (in which the bottle of pills is accidentally mislabeled). I hope that I also have shed some light on the nature of autonomous action and on the complexity of the subject matter.

In this article, I have had something to say about intentional action, voluntary action, free action, and autonomous action. In each of these spheres, one properly wonders how far one can move – along various dimensions – from seemingly paradigmatic instances of the kind of action at issue and still find instances of that kind of action. And in each sphere, one encounters difficult cases. Sometimes, it is difficult to make a confident judgment about whether a featured action is or is not intentional, voluntary, free, or autonomous – even when we know all the other relevant details about it. That is part of what keeps philosophers of action with a penchant for conceptual analysis in business. But we should be confident that when another agent's influence on your conduct benefits from his having surreptitiously seized something approaching complete control over whether you *A* or not – as in the case of King George raising property taxes by five percent – you are heteronomous in that connection and therefore do not autonomously *A*.[8]

## References

Aristotle. 1915. *Nicomachean Ethics*. Vol. 9 of William Ross, ed. *The Works of Aristotle*. London: Oxford University Press.
Arpaly, N. 2003. *Unprincipled Virtue*. New York: Oxford University Press.
Davidson, D. 1980. *Essays on Actions and Events*. Oxford: Clarendon Press.
Feinberg, J. 1986. *Harm to Self*. New York: Oxford University Press.
Fischer, J. 1994. *The Metaphysics of Free Will*. Cambridge, MA: Blackwell.
Fischer, J., and M. Ravizza. 1998. *Responsibility and Control: A Theory of Moral Responsibility*. New York: Cambridge University Press.
Fischer, J., and N. Tognazzini. 2009. The Truth About Tracing. *Noûs* 43: 531–556.
Frankfurt, H. 1988. *The Importance of What We Care About*. Cambridge: Cambridge University Press.
———. 2002. Reply to John Martin Fischer. In *Contours of Agency*, ed. S. Buss and L. Overton, 27–31. Cambridge, MA: MIT Press.
Ginet, C. 1990. *On Action*. Cambridge: Cambridge University Press.
Goldman, A. 1970. *A Theory of Human Action*. Englewood Cliffs: Prentice-Hall.
Killmister, S. 2013. Autonomy and False Beliefs. *Philosophical Studies* 164: 513–531.
McKenna, M. 2005. The Relationship Between Autonomous and Morally Responsible Agency. In *Personal Autonomy*, ed. J. Taylor, 205–234. Cambridge: Cambridge University Press.
———. 2012. *Conversation and Responsibility*. Oxford: Oxford University Press.
Mele, A. 1995. *Autonomous Agents: From Self-Control to Autonomy*. Oxford: Oxford University Press.
———. 2006. *Free Will and Luck*. New York: Oxford University Press.
———. 2009. Moral Responsibility and History Revisited. *Ethical Theory and Moral Practice* 12: 463–475.
———. 2010. Moral Responsibility for Actions: Epistemic and Freedom Conditions. *Philosophical Explorations* 13: 101–111.
Mele, A., and P. Moser. 1994. Intentional Action. *Noûs* 28: 39–68.
Thalberg, I. 1977. *Perception, Emotion, and Action*. New Haven: Yale University Press.
Thomson, J. 1977. *Acts and OtherEvents*. Ithaca: Cornell University Press.
Weimer, S. 2009. Beyond History: The Ongoing Aspects of Autonomy. *Journal of Ethics and Social Philosophy* 4: 1–31.

[8] I wrote this paper for a 2012 conference at the Centre for Advanced Study in Bioethics, University of Münster. I made some small changes while hiding out during the COVID-19 pandemic.

# Chapter 7
# How Much Understanding Is Needed for Autonomy?

**James Stacey Taylor**

**Abstract** How much understanding should be required of a person with respect to her actions and their implications for her to be autonomous with respect to her decisions to perform them? I defend a thin approach to the question of how much understanding of her acts a person should possess for her possibly to be autonomous with respect to her decisions to perform them: That a person could be autonomous with respect to her decision to perform a certain action if she understood both the nature of the act and its expected implications under the intensional description under which she intentionally performed it. This paper is divided into three sections. First, I argue that a concern for the moral value of autonomy does not undergird the ethical requirement to secure a person's informed consent to her medical treatment. Second, I respond to several objections that have been leveled against this argument that focus on its implicit premise that only a thin understanding of one's actions is required for one to be autonomous with respect to one's decisions to perform them. I conclude by indicating why this minimalist account of autonomy that I defend is preferable to its more robust competitors.

In his autobiographical work *Surely You're Joking Mr. Feynman* the Nobel-prize winning physicist Richard Feynman tells a story about an experience that he had as a consultant to an engineering project. Faced with a set of plans, he was unwilling to admit that he didn't know what some of the symbols for the parts were, and so he hit on an ingenious way to discover their meaning without admitting his ignorance. Pointing to one of the mysterious symbols, he asked "What would happen if that valve were left open?" expecting to be corrected as to the symbol's meaning. The engineers looked carefully at the plans, became visibly alarmed, and consulted among themselves, before thanking him profusely (and with great admiration!) for so quickly identifying a major flaw in the design of their system.

---

J. S. Taylor (✉)
The College of New Jersey, Ewing, NJ, USA
e-mail: jtaylor@tcnj.edu



J. F. Childress, M. Quante (eds.), *Thick (Concepts of) Autonomy*, Philosophical Studies Series 146, https://doi.org/10.1007/978-3-030-80991-1_7

Clearly, Feynman did not autonomously identify a flaw in the design of the valve system, for he had no understanding of what he was doing. He did not, in any meaningful sense, "direct himself" to decide to identify the flaw, as he might have done had he both understood the plans he was examining and the engineering principles involved. (Although he did "direct himself" to decide to point at a particular symbol, not knowing he was identifying a flaw.) To be autonomous with respect to a decision to perform a certain action, then, the person must understand what he is doing.[1] As such, it is not surprising that contemporary theories of autonomy have built into them the requirement that a person understand what she is doing for her to be autonomous with respect to her decisions (or her actions, or her effective first-order desires).[2] Thomas Beauchamp and James Childress, for example, make this requirement explicit when they hold that to be autonomous a person must act "with understanding" (Beauchamp and Childress 1994, 123). It is also implicit in Gerald Dworkin's (early) requirement that for a person to be autonomous with respect to a motivating desire she be procedurally independent with respect to it, and hence not subject to "manipulation, deception, the withholding of relevant information, and so on" (Dworkin 1976, 25).

Yet although there is widespread agreement that autonomy requires understanding there has been little discussion of how *much* a person should be required to understand her action and its implications for her to be autonomous with respect to her decision to perform it.[3] This oversight is surprising. It would seem that if an account of autonomy requires that a person understand her actions and their implications for her to be autonomous with respect to her decision to perform them then it should include an account of how much understanding is required for the sake of theoretical completeness.[4] Moreover, providing an account of how much a person should understand her actions and their implications for her to be autonomous with respect to her decisions to perform them would seem to be critical for persons who wish to draw on discussions of the nature and value of autonomy to address issues in applied ethics where this concept plays a central role. In bioethics, for example, it is held that persons should give their informed consent to their treatment, where

[1] This focus in this essay is on "local" models of autonomy, which provide an account of what it is for a person to be autonomous with respect to some particular mental state or act, rather than on "global" accounts, which focus on what it is to have a capacity for autonomy.

[2] Here, the focus will be on what it is for a person to be autonomous with respect to her decisions—although the arguments for the thin approach to the degree of understanding that is required can be reprised with suitable modifications to establish the degree of understanding required for a person to be autonomous with respect to her actions or her effective first-order desires.

[3] In this paper I am addressing the question of how much understanding a person must have of her actions and their implications for her to be autonomous with respect to decisions to perform them, and so when I write of a person's understanding of her actions this should be understood as encompassing their implications, also, since a person's understanding of these is required for her to understand the actions that she performs (or considers performing).

[4] Beauchamp and Childress do go some way in this direction, noting that the degree of understanding that is required will be context-dependent—although this is still merely the first step towards providing such an account (Beauchamp and Childress 1994, 123).

this requirement is intended to protect patient autonomy by ensuring that they adequately understand the options available to them—a vague requirement that immediately raises the question of the standard of adequacy required. A person's autonomous consent is similarly held to be both necessary and authoritative in business ethics—although there, there is little discussion of the need to secure the informed consent of (for example) the contracting parties.

How much understanding, then, should be required of a person with respect to her actions and their implications for her to be autonomous with respect to her decisions to perform them? One who adopted a thin approach to this question would hold that a person could be autonomous with respect to her decision to perform a certain action if she understood both the nature of the act and its expected implications under the intensional description under which she intentionally performed it. By contrast, one who adopted a thicker approach to this question would hold that a person could only be autonomous with respect to her decision to perform a certain action if she understood both the nature of the act and its expected implications under that intensional description of the act that would be held by someone who *adequately* understood these (where the adequacy conditions are to be specified). For example, a proponent of a thicker approach to this question might hold that a person could only be autonomous with respect to those of her actions that she performed under an intensional description of them that correctly identified the likelihood that they would achieve her ends in performing them.

In this paper I will defend a thin approach to the question of how much understanding of her acts a person should possess for her possibly to be autonomous with respect to her decisions to perform them. To this end it will be divided into three sections. First, I will outline an argument for the conclusion that a concern for the moral value of autonomy does not undergird the ethical requirement to secure a person's informed consent to her medical treatment. Second, I will then outline and respond to several objections that have been leveled against this argument that focus on its implicit premise that only a thin understanding of one's actions is required for one to be autonomous with respect to one's decisions to perform them. (The focus of this second section will be on defending the theoretical point that one need only have a thin understanding of one's actions for one possibly to be autonomous with respect to one's decisions to perform them, rather than on defending the conclusion of the argument concerning the foundations of informed consent in which this plays a role.) Of course, showing that the view that only a thin understanding of one's actions is necessary for one to be autonomous with respect to one's decisions to perform them can be *defended* does not thereby show that this should also be *accepted*. And, indeed, this view of the degree of understanding that is required for autonomy could be criticized on the grounds that it fails to capture the best intuitive understanding of what it is to be autonomous: That one is autonomous when one's decisions lead to one's actions instantiating one's will in the world. To respond to this challenge, I will offer some indication in the concluding section of this paper as to why the more minimalist account of autonomy that I defend is preferable to its more robust competitors.

## 7.1 Autonomy and Informed Consent

It is widely held that respect for the value of autonomy undergirds the doctrine of informed consent (see Beauchamp and Childress 1994, 142–146). To be autonomous a person must direct her own life, make her own decisions, and perform her own actions; to the extent that her life, decisions, and actions are under the control of another she thereby suffers from a diminution on her autonomy with respect to them.[5] Given this, for a person to be autonomous with respect to her medical decisions it should be she, and not her healthcare provider, who decides what course of treatment she is to pursue.[6] To the extent that a person's healthcare provider attempts to control her medical decisions through deliberately failing to disclose information about them to her, or through misrepresenting the risks and benefits of each to her, or through otherwise selectively presenting her with information in an attempt to guide her decisions, then, if he is successful in such manipulations, he will compromise her autonomy with respect to them. Hence, to ensure that healthcare professionals do not compromise the autonomy of their patients they should provide unbiased information about their treatment options to them. In requiring that they do this, then, the doctrine of informed consent appears to be grounded in the principle of respect for autonomy.

As will be outlined below, however, it is possible for a person to *fail* to give her informed consent to the course of treatment that she pursues, and yet still be fully autonomous with respect to her decision to pursue it, and the actions that she takes to do this. Since in many such cases it would still be appropriate to hold the healthcare professional who failed to secure his patient's informed consent to her course of treatment blameworthy for this failure, even though it did not adversely affect the patient's autonomy, it appears that the doctrine of informed consent rests on something other than a concern for the moral value of autonomy.[7]

How, then, could a person fail to give her informed consent to her treatment and yet still retain full autonomy with respect to her treatment decisions and consequent actions? The key to answering this question lies in recognizing that a person will be autonomous with respect to her decisions if it is she, and not someone else, who controls what it is that she decides to do. To see this, consider the case of Iago and Othello from Shakespeare's *Othello*. Through a series of manipulations and insinuations Iago convinces Othello that his wife is having an affair with his, Iago's, rival Cassio, which leads to Othello smothering her from jealousy. Here, the font of the decision for Othello to kill Desdemona was Iago, not Othello, and it is through

[5] This characterization of what it is to be autonomous is compatible with a wide variety of views of how much understanding of one's actions is necessary for one to be autonomous with respect to one's decisions to perform them.

[6] This claim is compatible with a person choosing to abdicate her decision to her healthcare provider, perhaps believing that he will make a better decision for her than she will.

[7] Many, but not necessarily all, cases. It might be that the healthcare provider inadvertently failed to secure his patients' informed consent to her treatment for a reason other than negligence that could be excused.

Iago's manipulation of Othello that he killed his wife. Since Othello was manipulated into making the decision to kill Desdemona by Iago, and hence it was not Othello himself, but Iago, who directed him do this, Othello's autonomy with respect to this decision was compromised.

The lesson to be learned from *Othello*—and that which makes it relevant to both discussions of the relationship between autonomy and informed consent, and discussions of the degree of understanding that is needed for a person to be autonomous with respect to her decisions—is that a person will suffer from compromised autonomy with respect to her decisions to act if they are controlled by another. Control is an intentionally characterized concept: A will only control the decisions of B if she intends so to do. To see this, consider a (non-existent) variant on *Othello*—*PseudoOthello*. In this version of the play PseudoIago's communications with PseudoOthello are precisely the same as they are in *Othello*, but with one crucial difference: In *PseudoOthello* PseudoIago engages in no manipulation at all, but simply descriptively provides PseudoOthello with the facts as he sees them, devoid of guile. Since in *PseudoOthello* it was PseudoOthello, and not PseudoIago, who was the font of PseudoOthello's (identical) decisions, Othello's autonomy with respect to them was uncompromised. Thus, given that the only differences between *Othello* and *PseudoOthello* are that in the former, but not the latter, Iago intended to usurp the direction of Othello's actions, and that in the former, but not the latter, Othello's autonomy was compromised as a result of his decisions being under the control of Iago, it is clear that a necessary condition (but not sufficient) for one person to control the decisions of another is that she intend so to do.

Let us now return to the question of the relationship between autonomy and informed consent—and hence to the question of how much understanding is needed for a person to be autonomous with respect to her decisions. Since a necessary condition for one person to control the decisions made by another is that she intend to do so a healthcare professional who deliberately withheld information from her patients to ensure that they made the decisions she wanted them to make (and was successful in her efforts so to do) would indeed be usurping their autonomy with respect to their decisions. However, a healthcare professional who *negligently* failed to provide her patients with sufficient information for them to make informed decisions concerning their treatments would *not* be intending to exercise control over the decisions that they made. As such, then, although her ill-informed patients would not have given their *informed* consent to their treatment decisions they would not have suffered from any diminution in their autonomy with respect to them. However, despite this, we would still blame the negligent healthcare professional for failing to secure her patients' informed consent to their treatment. And, since this is so, it appears that it is not concern for autonomy, but for something else, that undergirds the doctrine of informed consent, with autonomy being valued primarily for its use in enabling those who exercise it to secure this "something else" (see Taylor 2004).

## 7.2 Defending the Thin View of How Much Understanding is Needed for Autonomy

This account of why it is not the value of autonomy, but the value of "something else" that a person's exercise of autonomy might secure her, is of obvious interest to medical ethicists concerned with the ethical foundations of informed consent. But it is also of wider theoretical interest, for two reasons. First, this account of why it is not the value of autonomy that provides the ethical foundations for the requirement that a healthcare professional secure the informed consent of her patients to their treatment is based on a thin view of how much understanding of her actions a person must possess for her to be autonomous with respect to her decisions to perform them. A full defense of this revisionary account of the relationship between autonomy and informed consent would thus require a defense of the view that a person need only have a thin understanding of the acts that she performs for her to be fully autonomous with respect to them. Second, since the above argument held that a person's autonomy with respect to her decisions will be compromised if it is not she, but another, who controls what decisions she makes, and since it also held that control is an intentionally characterized concept, if the above argument is correct it entails that the question of whether a person is autonomous with respect to her acts cannot be decided only by reference to her own mental states. Instead, this question could only be decided by reference to both *her* mental states, *and* those of others, to ensure that her decision-making process is not under another's control. To put this colloquially, the above argument entails that whether or not *I* am autonomous with respect to my decisions to perform certain actions will depend in part on the mental states of *others*.

While the radically externalist implications of the above argument are striking, it is the thin understanding of autonomy that this argument is based on that has drawn the most criticism, with critics charging that this thin approach to understanding the degree of understanding that is required of a person to be autonomous with respect to her decisions is too impoverished. The aim of this section of the paper is thus to defend the thin view of the degree of understanding that a person must have for her to be autonomous with respect to her decisions, and consequent actions, that undergirded the above analysis of the relationship between autonomy and informed consent. In so doing the above view of the relationship between autonomy and informed consent will also be defended—although defending this is not the primary focus of this paper.

### 7.2.1 *The Objection from the Best Intensional Description*

The first objection to the thin account of how much understanding of her actions a person needs to be autonomous with respect to them that the above argument is based on begins with the claim that, occasionally, owing to the ignorance of the acting agent the intensional description under which she performs an action is not that which would best describe it from the point of view of a neutral third party. For example, while the description of Oedipus' act of marriage under which he performed it was "marrying Jocasta," an informed third party would hold that the most appropriate intensional description of this act would be "marrying his mother". Since owing to his lack of understanding of what he was doing that arose from his failing to perform his act under the intensional description that would be judged most appropriate for it by an informed third party, Oedipus suffered from a diminution in his autonomy with respect to it. He did not "direct himself" to perform the act that he actually performed, where the relevant intensional description of "the act that he actually performed" that should be used to assess this claim is that which would be deemed the most appropriate one by an informed third party. With this claim in hand, the proponent of this objection then notes that both Othello and PseudoOthello performed their deadly acts under the description "kill my unfaithful wife". However, since neither of their wives were actually unfaithful this would not be the most appropriate intensional description of their acts (instead, their acts would be more appropriately described by informed third party observers as "killing a faithful wife"), and so both of them would suffer from equally diminished autonomy with respect to their acts of smothering their wives.[8] Thus, the proponent of this objection concludes, it is clear that a thicker approach to the type of understanding that is required for a person to be autonomous with respect to her actions than that which underlies the above argument is required. And, moreover, since both Othello and PseudoOthello suffered from diminished autonomy with respect to their actions, and these diminutions are explicable in terms of their lack of understanding, rather than in terms of being subject to the control of another, the above argument concerning the relationship between autonomy and informed consent does not entail that one person's autonomy will crucially depend on the mental states of another.[9]

This objection is based on the view that an informed third party would judge that the acts of both Othello and PseudoOthello would be most appropriately described as "killing my unfaithful wife". But this act description is overly rich, for it contains both a description of the action and (implicitly) the reason why the act was done. In the context of this argument, however, it is only the (descriptive) *description of the act that is being performed* that is relevant, with the (normative) *reason for the performance of this action* being separable from this. What is of interest is whether Othello and PseudoOthello were autonomous with respect to the acts that they performed, not the separate issue of the reason why they performed those acts. Hence, only the description of the act is relevant. With this noted, the above objection can be revisited. It is not clear that the act-description "killing my unfaithful wife"

[8] Note that the claim that they suffered from diminished autonomy with respect to these acts is compatible with both the claim that they were nonautonomous with respect to them, and the (weaker) claim that while they were autonomous with respect to them, this was to a reduced degree.

[9] A version of this objection appeared in the original version of this paper; this (more robust) version was pressed on me by John Christman.

should be understood as being elliptical for the act-description "killing my wife because she is unfaithful". If this is so, then the most appropriate description of the actual act that is being performed will be "killing my wife" (with the adjective being indicative of the reason why this as done). Both Othello and PseudoOthello are thus performing the acts that they believe that they are performing; they are directing themselves to perform the acts (killing their wives) that they believe that they are performing. As such, then, *when their understanding of the acts that they are performing is alone considered*, they are fully autonomous with respect to them. It is only when we realize that Othello was subject to the control of Iago that we revise our assessment of the degree to which he was autonomous with respect to the smothering of Desdemona.

To support this response to the above objection consider a third case—OutsourceOthello. In this example, Othello hires an assassin to smother Desdemona, which the assassin duly does. The assassin has been hired to "kill an unfaithful wife", just as both Othello and PseudoOthello aimed "to kill my unfaithful wife". Like Othello and PseudoOthello, then, this assassin performs an action without understanding that he was not killing an unfaithful wife. However, despite this it would be implausible to hold that the assassin's autonomy with respect to his killing of Desdemona was impaired in any way because of this. And the reason for this is because one can distinguish between "killing a wife" and "killing an unfaithful wife", with the latter description of the act being both a description of the act itself ("killing a wife") and an account of why this was done ("because she was unfaithful"). Thus, the mere fact that the assassin did not succeed in killing an unfaithful wife does not undermine the fact that (like Othello and PseudoOthello) he achieved what he set out to do—namely, kill Desdemona. A proponent of the above objection might respond at this point by claiming that the assassin was fully autonomous with respect to his acts as he did not care whether Desdemona was unfaithful or not, whereas Othello and PseudoOthello did. Thus, since they failed to achieve what they intended to achieve by killing Desdemona whereas as the assassin achieved what he set out to do, they suffer from diminished autonomy with respect to their murderous acts in a way that he does not. But this response to the above defense offered against this first objection confuses a person's being autonomous with respect to her action with her achieving what she set out to achieve by performing it. A person (such as, here, Othello and PseudoOthello) could be perfectly autonomous with respect to her acts even if her performance of them does not achieve what she intended, and so her exercise of her autonomy has little instrumental value for her. But that this is so does not undermine the thin approach to the degree of understanding that a person needs to be autonomous with respect to her actions. Indeed, this should be clear from the fact that the observation that a person's act might have little instrumental value for her is perfectly in accord with the original analysis of the relationship between autonomy and informed consent: a person might be fully autonomous with respect to her medical decisions, but, owing to negligence by her healthcare provider, these decisions might fail to lead he to achieve what she intended to achieve. They would thus have low instrumental value for here, and it is on this basis that is, on the basis of the failure to secure the value that she was attempting to exercise her autonomy to secure—that we would hold her negligent healthcare provider to be morally culpable for his failure to secure her informed consent.

### 7.2.2 *Agency, Autonomy, and Understanding*

The objection that the thin view of the degree to which a person must understand her actions to be autonomous with respect to her decisions to perform them is mistaken because it fails to recognize that both Othello and PseudoOthello suffered from diminished autonomy with respect to their acts of killing their wives can thus be met. But this view of the degree to which a person must understand her actions to be autonomous with respect to decisions to perform them faces a second serious objection: That it lacks the conceptual resources to distinguish between (mere) agents and autonomous agents.

It is widely accepted that small children and cognitively impaired adults are not autonomous agents.[10] However, both children and cognitively impaired adults can satisfy the thin view of the degree of understanding of their actions and their implications that is necessary for them to be autonomous with respect to their decisions to perform those actions: They decide to perform acts under particular intensional descriptions, and understand (to a degree) the implications of their actions. As such, then, a proponent of the thin view of the degree to which a person must understand her actions to be autonomous with respect to her decisions to perform them seems committed to endorsing the implausible claim that small children and cognitively impaired adults are autonomous with respect to their decisions to perform their actions.[11]

But while this objection is initially plausible it is based on confusing the necessary conditions required for an agent to be autonomous with respect to her decisions and those that are sufficient for this. Clearly, it is necessary for an agent to be autonomous with respect to her decisions that she possesses the thin understanding of the actions and their implications that she decides to perform. But more is also needed. In particular, for an agent to be autonomous with respect to a decision that she makes she must have made that decision "as a result of a decision-making procedure that she is satisfied with as being her decision-making procedure for making the type of decision that is in question" (Taylor 2009, 8).[12] Since being satisfied with a

[10] Widely, but not universally (see Mullin 2007).

[11] I thank Jessica Flannigan for pressing a version of this objection.

[12] This "Degree Condition" for autonomy is supplemented by both a Threshold Condition and a Tracing Condition to provide an account of "practical autonomy" (Taylor 2009, 6–11). Note that as it was explicated in *Practical Autonomy and Bioethics* this account of practical autonomy is incomplete. This is because, in brief, it held that a person would be autonomous with respect to her decision to perform a certain action if the information on which she based her decision had not been affected in some way without her knowledge by another with the aim of leading her to make

decision-making procedure requires that one have reflected upon it and accepted it as one's own, this additional requirement for a person to be autonomous with respect to her decisions will preclude small children and cognitively impaired adults being autonomous with respect to their decisions—even if they understood their actions and their implications to the minimal degree required by the thin view of the degree of such understanding that is required.

### 7.2.3 Maclean's Objections

The final objection against the thin view of understanding that undergirded the above argument that will be considered here has been developed by Alaisdair Maclean. Writing of the example of Iago and Othello, Maclean argues

> This example, while superficially attractive, fails to acknowledge a crucial issue. That is: whose responsibility was it to ensure that Othello was sufficiently informed to make the decision? If the duty is Othello's then his capacity for autonomy has not been compromised because it is his responsibility, and not Iago's, to ensure that he is sufficiently well-informed; Iago has done nothing that would constrain Othello's ability to satisfy himself that the information is sufficient and reliable. However, if the duty is Iago's, and it is reasonable for Othello to rely on the information, then Othello's autonomy has been compromised because he has been caused to believe that he is sufficiently informed (Maclean 2009, 43).

Noting that in modern society "it is impossible to live without relying on information provided by experts," Maclean continues,

> Where the expert has a duty to provide sufficient information… then any failure to do so, whether intended or not, will lead to a false reliance that undermines the individual's autonomy. By inducing a false belief in the patient, that he or she knows enough to make a rational decision, the patient's motivation for seeking additional information is removed. Thus, although the patient is free to seek additional information, he or she falsely believes there is no reason to do so… This means that where a physician… misinforms the patient this reduces the patient's ability to make a rational—and hence autonomous—decision (Maclean 2009, 43 – 44).

Although it is not completely clear, Maclean's argument seems to be this: (1) That if B is responsible for ensuring that he was sufficiently informed then, if A does not

a particular decision, or particular type of decision, or, if it had, she was aware of how it had been so affected (the Threshold Condition), and if she was satisfied that the decision-making procedure that she used to make the decision in question was that which she was satisfied with in making decisions of that type (the Degree Condition). But this account allows the possibility that a person could be manipulated into being satisfied with a decision making procedure that she used to make a decision D when she normally would not be satisfied with that procedure in making a decision of type D. And if such manipulation was done with the intent of her making a particular decision D without admitting the possibility that she would revise her decision then she would not be autonomous with respect to D. Given this possibility, the original Threshold Condition must be modified, so that it applies not only to the information on which the person in question bases her decision about whether or not to do X, but also to the information that the persons' satisfaction with her decision is based upon. I thank Steve Weimer for pressing me on this point.

constrain his ability to do so, B's capacity for autonomy has not been compromised, and so the thin view of how much understanding is required of B concerning her acts is sufficient for her to be autonomous with respect to her decisions to perform them; (2) That if A has a duty to ensure that B was sufficiently well-informed such that if he fails to do so B's autonomy will be compromised, then (if it would be reasonable for B to rely on A) the thin view of how much understanding is required of B concerning her acts is not sufficient for her to be autonomous with respect to her decisions to perform them (for the thin view does not require that a person be sufficiently informed for her to be fully autonomous with respect to her decisions); (3) A physician has a duty to ensure that her patients are sufficiently well-informed about their treatment options, and so (from (2) and (3)); (4) the thin view of how much understanding is required of A concerning her acts is not sufficient for her to be autonomous with respect to her decisions to perform them in a medical context.

While Maclean's immediate conclusion is that "Taylor's argument fails to sever the connection between [informed] consent and autonomy" his argument also supports the more general claim that at least in some cases a person's having only a thin understanding of her actions is insufficient for her to be autonomous with respect to her decisions to perform them. Yet there is no reason to accept either of these conclusions. As is clear from the above reconstruction of Maclean's argument his conclusion rests on premises (2) and (3); (1) is redundant (for it allows that the thin approach to the degree of understanding that is required for a person to be autonomous with respect to her acts is acceptable, at least under some circumstances).[13] And the core of each of these two premises as they pertain to the question of how much understanding a person must have concerning her actions for her to be autonomous with respect to her decisions to make them is the question of whether or not she is "sufficiently informed". But there's the rub—for this raises the question of what criterion should be used to determine whether or not a person is "sufficiently informed". The criterion clearly cannot be that the person is sufficiently informed to be autonomous with respect to her decisions to perform the acts that she does, since the underlying issue is precisely what degree of information (and hence understanding) is required for her to possess this property with respect to them. That is, one cannot reject the thin view of the relationship between a person's autonomy with respect to her decisions and her understanding of her actions on the grounds that it would hold a person to be autonomous with respect to her decisions even if she was

[13] This is a good thing for Maclean, for there are two problems with his first premise, both in itself and when conjoined with the example of Iago and Othello. First, the question is not whether A's capacity for autonomy (i.e., his ability to be autonomous) would be compromised by the degree to which he understands his actions and their implications, but whether the degree to which he understands them is sufficient for him to be autonomous with respect to them. This, however, might be merely a semantic issue, and there will be no violence done to the premise if this were changed. However, when Maclean applies this premise to the case of Iago and Othello he claims that Iago did not constrain Othello's ability to ensure that he was sufficiently well-informed about his situation. This claim is either straightforwardly mistaken (for the very point of *Othello* is to show how Iago manipulates Othello) or else Maclean has an implausibly restricted view of what would count as one person's constraining another.

insufficiently informed about her actions properly to be so, since this would clearly beg the question against the proponent of the thin view.

A more charitable interpretation of Maclean's argument here, then, would hold that the question of whether a person is "sufficiently informed" should be assessed against something other than her autonomy. What, then, should this be? Recall here that Maclean holds that "…where a physician… misinforms the patient this reduces the patient's ability to make a rational—and hence autonomous—decision" (Maclean 2009, 44). As written, this is mistaken on two counts: A person can make perfectly rational decisions on the basis of poor or false information, and there is (outside the Kantian tradition) no necessary link between autonomy and rationality (see Double 1992; Noggle 1997). Perhaps, though, what Maclean means here is not that a misinformed person cannot make a rational decision, but that she cannot make an *advisable* decision (see Gibbard 1998, 19). If this interpretation of what Maclean intends here is correct then the question of whether a person is sufficiently informed will become the question of whether she has sufficient information to decide to perform that act which is likely to achieve the ends that she intends to achieve through its performance. But if this is how we are to understand Maclean's view here it will face the response that was offered to the final defense of the Objection from the Best Intensional Description—that we can distinguish between a person's being autonomous with respect to her decisions and the acts that she performs as a result of them, and her making good instrumental use of her autonomy. Fortunately for Maclean, it seems that this is not how we should understand his view. This is because Maclean allows that a person who performs an action that is *not* advisable for her could still be fully autonomous with respect to her decision to perform it provided that it was *her* responsibility to ensure that she was sufficiently well-informed prior to making it. As such, then, the fact that B decided to perform an action that was inadvisable for her does not ground Maclean's view that she thereby suffered from diminished autonomy. Perhaps, then, Maclean's view is that B suffers from a diminution in her autonomy with respect to her (inadvisable) decision as a result of her ceding control to A over the decision as to when she would be sufficiently well-informed to decide which act to perform, and his subsequent misuse of this control. But this cannot be Maclean's view, either. For Maclean, B does not suffer from a diminution in autonomy with respect to her ceding this control to A for if A were to perform his duty and provide her with adequate information—and so Maclean's objection is not based on B's ceding control to A. The final possible interpretation of Maclean's view is that B will suffer a diminution in her autonomy if she cedes control to A *and* A subsequently misinforms her, thus leading her to make an inadvisable decision. But it would be odd if this were Maclean's view, for it is difficult to see how the combination of B's ceding control and making an inadvisable decision would compromise her autonomy when neither would do so alone. Maclean, then, has no way of explaining why the issue of who is responsible for informing B is so "crucial" to the question of whether or not B was autonomous with respect to her decisions and consequent actions. There is thus no reason to accept the argument that Maclean offers that supports the claim that at least in some cases the thin view of the relationship between a person's having only a thin understanding of her actions is insufficient for her to be autonomous with respect to her decisions to perform them.

## 7.3 Conclusion

In David Lodge's academic satire *Changing Places* one of the characters, an American careerist academic called Professor Zapp, was described as disliking English academics, in part as they spent all their time complaining about the American academy while at the same time freeloading off it as much as they could, and in part because they seemed to consider their job complete if they raised questions about issues rather than actually answering them. In concluding this essay I am sure that I, too, would annoy Professor Zapp, for this paper comes in the middle of a research project, rather than at its end—and so no doubt there remain questions to be asked to which I have not provided any answers. Before looking forward to such annoyance, however, it is time to take stock of the positive conclusions that can be drawn from the above discussion. First, the thin view of the degree of understanding of her actions and their implications that a person must possess for her to be autonomous with respect to her decision to perform them can be defended against the objections outlined above: the objection from the best intensional description, the objection that it failed to distinguish between non-autonomous and autonomous agents, and Maclean's objections. Second, while the account of autonomy discussed in this paper is based on a thin view of the degree of understanding that a person must have of her actions to be autonomous with respect to her decision to perform them it is, in another respect, a very thick view of autonomy indeed, insofar as the answer to the question of whether a person is autonomous with respect to her decisions will depend not only upon her mental states, but on those of others. But while it might at first sight render this account of autonomy implausible (for it might seem odd that *my* autonomy depends in part on the mental states *of others*) the fact that this is an externalist, relational account of autonomy is a strength. The question of when a person is autonomous with respect to her decisions is the question of when it is she, and not someone else, who is the font of them. Unlike the property of identification (which is a metaphysical property ascribed to persons with respect to those of their effective first-order desires that are truly her own, that can be properly attributed to her as a person), autonomy (at least as it is understood above) is a *political* property, one that persons have or lack on the basis of their relationships with other persons (see Taylor 2009, chapter 3). Thus, since control is an intentionally characterized concept, and so one can only answer the question of whether person one person controlled the decisions of another by reference to the first person's mental states, it is only to be expected that the question of whether a person is autonomous with respect to her decisions must be answered by reference to the mental states of others.[14]

It is now time to annoy Professor Zapp. It was argued above that autonomy only requires persons to have a thin understanding of their actions for them to be autonomous with respect to their decisions to perform them. The intuitive basis for this argument was that a person was autonomous with respect to his decisions if was she, and not someone else, who directed her to make them. But it must be admitted that this is not the only way in which one might intuitively understand autonomy.[15] One might hold that a person was autonomous with respect to her decisions if they led her to perform actions that enabled her to instantiate her will in the world. On this understanding of autonomy having only a thin understanding of one's actions and their implications would be insufficient for a person to be autonomous with respect to her decisions to perform them, for this would be unlikely to enable one to instantiate her will through her actions. A person, for example, whose physician negligently failed to inform her of some of the serious implications of her treatment would not be able effectively to instantiate her will in the world, for she would lack the requisite information to do so.[16]

Which of these intuitive understandings of autonomy should take precedence? Although this issue cannot be conclusively settled here it should be noted that there is at least *prima facie* reason to prefer the thinner approach to autonomy defended above. First, the proponents of the more robust understanding of autonomy cannot criticize its thinner rival simply by noting that this account of autonomy appears to be of little value. One might, for example, note that the thinner account of autonomy

[14]As part of his argument against the thin account of understanding that a person must have of her actions and their implications in order for her to be autonomous with respect to her decision to perform them, Maclean argues that control should not be understood as an intentionally characterized concept, and that one person could exercise control over the actions of another without thereby intending to do so. In support of this view he offers an example in which children inadvertently switch train tracks from one line to another, and thus "undermined the railway company's control of the train's route"; an example, he believes, whereby one party's control is undermined unintentionally by another. But this example fails to show that control can be exercised unintentionally, for the children do not control the direction that the train goes in; they merely affect it. To see the distinction here, consider the difference between a leaf's being blown by the wind as it falls, and its being choreographed in its falling by someone with a radio-controlled device whose receiver and engine she has attached to the leaf, so that it will weave the patterns that she desires as it descends. Here, the wind would not control where or how the leaf falls, but would merely affect this; the person with the radio-controlled device, however, would control it, and not merely affect it, for she would intentionally direct its falling. More generally, note that Maclean's example here fails to touch the examples of *Othello* and *Pseudo Othello*, for the childrens' switching of the tracks does not affect (and so cannot control) the decisions of the railway company's personnel; nor does it affect (and hence does not control) their actions. Instead, they merely affect (but do not control) the outcomes of these decisions and actions. As such, Maclean's example is irrelevant to the Shakespearian examples which focus on establishing that for one person to control the decisions (and hence actions) of another she must intend to do so, for it does not address this point at all.

[15]Although it might be that this would still be the most defensible approach, as is indicated below.

[16]This appears to be the understanding of autonomy that Mele accepts at times (Mele 1995, 180, 181).

would hold that a person could be fully autonomous with respect to her decision to perform some action that owing to her ignorance of its true nature would not only fail to advance her interests, but would actively hinder them. With this observation in hand, one might then note that it is not clear why one should value being "autonomous" in this sense. Hence, one might conclude, since the possession of autonomy is supposed to be valuable, then insofar as its possession is not (obviously) valuable when it is understood thinly thinner conceptions should be rejected.[17] But this objection moves too quickly, for (as noted above, in response to the Objection from the Best Intensional Description) a proponent of the thinner understanding of autonomy defended here can readily distinguish between a persons' being autonomous with respect to her decisions *simpliciter* and the degree to which her autonomy is of instrumental value to her (Taylor, 2009, chapter 10). And, with this distinction in hand, she could then argue that the value of autonomy was primarily instrumental, such that while a person could be fully autonomous with respect to those of her decisions that were made in conditions of relative ignorance (for she need only have a thin understanding of her actions and their implications for her to be autonomous with respect to her decisions to make them) her autonomy would possess only low (or no) value under such circumstances. Second, while the more minimalist account of autonomy can respond to the charge that it cannot account for the value of autonomy the proponents of its more robust rival face a problem of vagueness, for it is not clear what would count as "instantiating one's will in the world". Obviously, requiring that a person's actions must lead her to succeed in her goals for her to count as being autonomous with respect to her decisions to perform them would be an implausibly stringent standard. But some degree of success in a person's decisions leading to her achieving her goals must be required for her to be autonomous with respect to them on this more robust account of autonomy, for unless this is so it is unclear how one is to understand the claim that to be autonomous a person must instantiate her will in the world.[18] Given the vagueness of this more robust approach to understanding autonomy, and given the fact that the thinner account defended above can account for the view that in some cases a person's autonomy will be of little value, there is at least *prima facie* reason to accept the thinner account. As such, then, the simple answer to the question of how much understanding is required for autonomy is: Very little.[19]

---

[17] This criticism of the thin account of how much understanding is necessary for autonomy is similar to that which Berlin (Berlin 1969, 124) recognizes could be leveled against the negative account of freedom.

[18] A weaker requirement might be that a person is autonomous with respect to her decisions only if it is likely that they will lead to her will being instantiated in the world. But while this might be a more plausible version of the more robust approach to autonomy, this plausibility comes at the cost of even more vagueness is its application.

[19] An earlier version of this paper was presented at the "Thick Concepts of Autonomy Conference" at the Center for Advanced Study of Bioethics, Westfalische-Wilhelms-Universität, Münster, Germany, October 2012. I thank all of the participants in that programme for their *exceptionally* helpful comments on my paper which helped me to improve it greatly.

## References

Beauchamp, Tom L., and James F. Childress. 1994. *Principles of Biomedical Ethics*. 4th ed. New York: Oxford University Press.

Berlin, Isaiah. 1969. Two Concepts of Liberty. In *Four Essays on Liberty*, ed. Isaiah Berlin, 118–172. Oxford: Oxford University Press. 124.

Double, Richard. 1992. Two Types of Autonomy Accounts. *Canadian Journal of Philosophy* 22 (1): 65–80.

Dworkin, Gerald. 1976. Autonomy and Behavior Control. *Hastings Center Report* 6 (1): 23–28.

Gibbard, Alan. 1998. *Wise Choices, Apt Feelings: A theory of normative judgment*. Oxford: Clarendon Press.

Maclean, Alasdair. 2009. *Autonomy, Informed Consent and Medical Law: A Relational Challenge*. Cambridge: Cambridge University Press.

Mele, Al. 1995. *Autonomous Agents: From Self-Control to Autonomy*. New York: Oxford University Press.

Mullin, Amy. 2007. Children, Autonomy, and Care. *Journal of Social Philosophy* 38 (4): 536–553.

Noggle, Robert. 1997. The Public Conception of Autonomy and Critical Self-Reflection. *Southern Journal of Philosophy* 34 (4): 495–515.

Taylor, James Stacey. 2004. Autonomy and Informed Consent: A Much Misunderstood Relationship. *Journal of Value Inquiry* 38 (3): 383–391.

———. 2009. *Practical Autonomy and Bioethics*. New York: Routledge.

# Chapter 8
# Is "Autonomy Talk" Misleading?

**Thomas Gutmann**

**Abstract** Especially during the last three decades, there has been a fine-grained debate on the notion of personal autonomy. This article will suggest taking one important distinction within this debate more seriously: the differentiation between (a) "personal autonomy" designating a family of ideal, gradual, and hence at least moderately perfectionist conceptions about what an autonomous person is and (b) what is called "autonomy as right" (Feinberg. 1986. 47). These are not different dimensions of one concept, but independent concepts with disparate, even conflicting normative functions and should be kept clearly separate from each other. Treating these two concepts merely as different aspects of one and the same notion of personal autonomy, as done by most authors, is severely misleading. For clarity, we will ultimately need different words for divergent concepts. It will be suggested that "autonomy as (moral or legal) right" should no longer be called "autonomy", but forthrightly the "right to self-determination" or, in accordance with Thomas Hobbes, "authority".

## 8.1 A Functional Approach

Autonomy—the question of whether a person is autonomous or acts autonomously or has the authority to act as she likes—has different functions in particular normative settings. One of the basic functions of autonomy—not only in bioethics and (medical) law—is related to a person's claim (her moral or legal right) to be respected as an agent entitled to choose her own path and follow it. "Autonomy as right" is what is meant when the "principle of respect for autonomy" is invoked in the way Beauchamp and Childress use the term in their *Principles of Biomedical*

T. Gutmann (✉)
Faculty of Law, University of Muenster, Muenster, Germany
e-mail: t.gutmann@uni-muenster.de



J. F. Childress, M. Quante (eds.), *Thick (Concepts of) Autonomy*, Philosophical Studies Series 146, https://doi.org/10.1007/978-3-030-80991-1_8

*Ethics* in regard to "individuals' decision-making": "To respect autonomous agents is to acknowledge their right to hold views, to make choices, and to take actions based on their values and beliefs" (Beauchamp and Childress 2013, 101 et seq., 106; cf. Beauchamp 2005). The necessarily formal notion of having a set of rights expressive of one's sovereignty over oneself (i.e. of having a protected space in which one may choose freely between options for action [Sect. 6][1]) may well be called a 'thin' concept of autonomy, as there is no specific content required for the choices such an autonomous (sovereign) person is allowed to make within such a right.[2] So where we have reason to conceive "autonomy as right" (i.e. as right of "self-determination" or as "authority", respectively), 'thick' concepts of autonomy are out of place.

## 8.2 'Thick' Concepts of Autonomy as Concepts of the Good Life

When I think about what kind person I want my 15-year old son to be or to become, what comes to my mind are so-called 'thick' concepts of autonomy referring to a certain personality structure.

I want him to be his own person, to live his life according to reasons, motives, and principles that are his own and thus give meaning and coherence to his life. I want him to have the second-order capacity to reflect critically upon his first-order preferences, desires, wishes, and so forth, and the capacity to identify with these or to attempt to change them in light of his higher-order preferences and values (Dworkin 1988, 20, 108; see Quante 2011, 598; id. 2017, 119 et seq.).[3] I want him to be authentic in the sense that he is able to reflectively endorse (or at least not be alienated from) his basic organizing values, motivations, and commitments in the

[1] The metaphor of space was always crucial for the notion of autonomy rights, see e.g. Feinberg 1986, 28, speaking of the "*sovereign authority* to govern oneself, which is absolute within one's own moral boundaries (one's 'territory', 'realm', 'sphere', or 'domain')"; Wellmann 1985, 95 ("dominion") and Steiner 1994, 90 ("domain"). The metaphor goes back at least to von Savigny 1867, 6, who (in this regard following) Immanuel Kant's notion of right) defines "the right in a subjective sense" as "a territory in which his will rules and rules with our consent". It was taken up in consequentialist accounts of (quasi-) rights to self-determination, see Mill 1992, Ch. I, IV ("Over himself, over his own body and mind, the individual is sovereign").

[2] Autonomy as right does not have to be exclusively a negative right. It may also generate reasons for others to assist or to promote the autonomy competence of others as well, cf. Beauchamp, Childress 2013, 101 et seq., and Mackenzie 2008. See for the needs of vulnerable persons who are attempting to *reconstruct* a sense of practical identity required for their autonomy, Christman 2014.

[3] Quante, in order to avoid a utopian ideal of autonomy that is unattainable for mortals, convincingly introduces a capacity for critical self-evaluation which contains a counterfactual: "a person has personal autonomy with respect to a first-order-attitude if she would be able to exercise the capacities necessary for personal autonomy if she noticed this first-order-attitude (or if someone asked her to critically reflect her first-order attitude)." Thus, permanent critical reflection and identification is not required for personal autonomy. Cf. Quante 2017, 119, 131, and also Christman's (2009, 155) hypothetical reflection condition for the authenticity element of autonomy.

light of his diachronic practical identity, i.e. the historical processes (including my own role in them) that gave rise to these characteristics (Christman 2009, 133 et seq., 143). I therefore hope that he will be able to evaluate the formation of his desires (Elster 1983, 109 et seqq.) in a process of sustained critical reflection (Christman 2009, 152), exercising the repertory of necessary skills for autonomous self-discovery and self-definition (Meyers 1989, 49; id. 2000, 163, 166). I want him to fully develop the affective attitudes—attitudes of self-respect, self-trust, and self-esteem—necessary for a view of himself as the legitimate source of reasons for acting (Mackenzie 2008, 524–527; Honneth and Anderson 2005). I want him to work through his unconscious connections of instinctual drives to a conscious liberty with which he can have his self-powers at his disposal as unimpededly as possible, without being hindered by frustrating, infantile expectations later in his life (Freud 1972a, 317; id. 1972b, 516; cf. Berofsky 1995). I want him to be responsive to a sufficiently wide range of reasons concerning his choices (Berofsky 1995, 182 et seq., 199) and to subject his opinions and tastes to rational scrutiny. I want him to be authentic to the extent that he can and does alter his convictions for these reasons of his own and that he does this without guilt or anxiety (Feinberg 1986, 33).

I want him to be programmatically autonomous, posing and answering the question "How do I want to live my life?" (Meyers 2004, 8; id. 1989), and, therefore, I would like him to lead a life that forms an ongoing narrative, a life with a high degree of biographical consistence and coherence which follows what Rawls calls a "rational life plan" that "would be chosen … with full deliberative rationality, that is, with full awareness of the relevant facts and after careful consideration of the consequences" (Rawls 1971, § 63, 408). In this sense, I want him to be a self-governing, planning agent (Bratman 1987; id. 2007, 195 et seq.), but, on the other hand, I do not want him to experience himself as a "tight identity knot" (Meyers 2000, 163), but to be able to seriously imagine alternative lives (Mackenzie 2000; Meyers 2004, 10) and to realize that this dynamic process of autonomous self-discovery and self-definition will be a lifelong journey based on piecemeal change, on improvisation, and on constant balancing of ambivalent and contradicting constituents of his identity (cf. Meyers 2000, 173–175).

Finally, I want him, on the basis of an authentic interpretation of his "real" objectives, to be able to make "strong" evaluations in regard to the success of his life and to his identity as a whole (Taylor 1985a, b; cf. Benn 1976, 125 et seq.; id. 1988, 9, 178 et seq.). However, in contrast to Taylor's overboarding 1980s communitarianism, I also want my son to free himself from unreasonable conformist attitudes and role expectations (Meyers 1989; id. 2000; Oshana 2006a; id. 2006b), as well from cognitive limitations on his spontaneous experience (Berofsky 1995). In other words, I want him to guide his life from his own perspective, rather than be manipulated by others, and to be able to free himself from "heterarchy" (Benn 1988, 164 et seqq.) and from considerations, values, desires, and emotions imposed externally upon him. I want him to have a "desire … for self-governance" (Oshana 2006a, 101), and yes, I even want him to be that kind of idiosyncratic eccentric John Stuart Mill associated with genius, mental vigour, and moral courage (Mill 1992, Ch. III). The latter being a little close to a specific male and atomistic fantasy, I do hope that all this will not prevent him from experiencing himself as deeply socially embedded, his capacity to exercise his autonomy depending (up to a certain point) on social institutions and the fragile nexus of relationships of trust, loyalty, friendship, love, caring, and shared values.[4]

I want all this because I care for what I think constitutes a good life for him. All these 'thick' notions of autonomy are different conceptions of the same concept of autonomy (and, although the variety of these conceptions demonstrates substantive philosophical disagreements about the conditions and capacities necessary for 'thick' autonomy, we do not have to choose between them here[5]). This concept of autonomy, however, is a concept of what it is to lead a 'good', valuable and flourishing life (Mackenzie 2008, 529).[6] Or at least, as long as the criteria for personal autonomy remain largely formal and are therefore not sufficient for a comprehensive definition of the good life (Quante 2017, 125), they still define a part of such a concept. As an ideal, the notion of autonomy used to qualify the structure of a person's life belongs to the realm of value-centered reasons (Benn 1988, 10). 'Thick' concepts of autonomy describe a value, even "an irrefutable" one (Christman 2015, Sub 1). Values can be realized more or less, which is one difference between values and rules.

## 8.3 The Good and the Right

One basic function of the notion of "autonomy"—not only in (bio-) ethics and (medical) law—, however, has to do not with the good, but with the right, and, as we shall see, with the idea of the priority of right (Rawls 1988). The latter is related to a person's claim (to her moral or legal right) to be respected as an agent who is entitled to choose her own conception of the good and follow it. To quote Rawls, persons are "self-authenticating sources of valid claims" (Rawls 2001, 23 et seq.) because identifying a natural person as a moral (or legal) person is to recognize her as a bearer of rights (Benn 1988, 9).

This realm of rights (cf. Thomson 1990) to self-determination is a central feature of our concept of normativity and deeply embedded in our normative (moral and legal) practices. In a sense, respect for persons may simply be respect for their rights

---

[4]Although, strictly speaking, some aspects of such a notion of "relational autonomy" (cf. Mackenzie and Stoljar 2000a) are no longer a concept of autonomy at all, but of aspects of human flourishing that should be clearly distinguished from personal autonomy.

[5]We can also skip the question here of whether "the ideal of personal autonomy […] requires not merely the presence of options, but of acceptable ones" (Raz 1986, 205) or "calls for positive freedom", "de facto power", and the social, political, and economically means to realize one's choices (Oshana 2006a, 101 et seq.; id. 2006b, 2; id. 1998; Mackenzie and Stoljar 2000a; Mackenzie 2014, 25).

[6]In a wider sense, personal autonomy in this sense is also one of the elements of well-being (cf. Mill 1992, Ch. III).

and their capacity to assert claims (Feinberg 1970). How central it is depends, of course, on the normative framework we (have reasons to) choose. For what we can call mainstream liberal Kantianism in moral and legal philosophy, respecting rights is the core element of morality which deals with what we owe to each other. It is a normative relation of (at least prima facie) lexical priority (Dworkin 1977). For a consequentialist, rights may be of only instrumental value for individual and collective well-being (Raz 1986, 185 et seq., 203 et seq.), and, for a principlist approach, the principle of respect for autonomy (i.e., for the right to self-determination) does not necessarily always have priority over other considerations (Beauchamp and Childress 2013, 101, 141).

Axel Honneth is right in pointing out that respecting rights is *one* basic form of social *recognition* and that it is the *only egalitarian* one (Honneth 1996, 109 "legal recognition"; cf. Honneth and Anderson 2005, 138). Being a moral and legal agent with free will, able to freely decide which actions to take and which path to follow in our life, applies to all of us equally. It is a conception of persons as moral equals. There is no *degree* of being worthy of this kind of recognition,[7] neither is there any room for exceptions or privileges. Law, at least in the Western legal tradition, is deeply embedded in this sort of egalitarian normative individualism, but for the purpose of this article, it suffices to address the right to self-determination as a moral claim.

## 8.4 Ideal and Threshold Concepts of Autonomy: Equality and Inclusion

In almost all the varieties of its philosophical use as described above (sub 2), a substantial concept of personal autonomy (autonomy$_i$) designates an ideal[8] which real persons can, at best, only approach. Autonomy in this sense is always a matter of degree—a person can be more or less autonomous (Mackenzie and Stoljar 2000b, 18). As a goal to be attained, "it may well be enjoyed by very few if any individuals" (Christman 2015, Sub 1.1.). In this development-orientated and thus broadly perfectionist sense, however, autonomy cannot be an essential condition for guaranteeing persons areas of liberty for self-responsible decision-making.

"Autonomy as right" (or better, the right of "self-determination") means that we attribute to individuals the normative competence for decisions concerning their own sphere of life (and corresponding duties for other persons at least not to interfere). Autonomy as the *ontic status* of being a person that can claim a right to self-determination (autonomy$_r$) must be independent of the question of how far she

[7] Cf. Darwall's (1977) notion of "recognition respect", which is neither context dependent nor a matter of degree.

[8] It may be "at best only a partial ideal"(Feinberg 1986, 45), "an actually unattainable ideal" (Quante 2017, 130) and "an ideal deeply rooted in the liberal tradition" (Benn 1988, 10), but it is an ideal.

realizes the value of autonomous personhood (autonomy$_i$). Therefore, when we address "autonomy as right" (autonomy$_r$) it is only a "threshold conception of natural competence—minimal relevant capacity for a task—that [must be] used in stipulations of necessary and sufficient conditions for the sovereign right of self-government ascribed to individuals" (Feinberg 1986, 29 et seq; Wikler 1983; VanDeVeer 1986, 351; Benn 1988, 10; Beauchamp 2005, 316). In order to be considered a valid decision-making body in one's own affairs, it must suffice to be sufficiently autonomous, i.e. to have basic cognitive and volitional competence (regarding rationality, self-control, and the absence of certain mental pathologies).[9] We have to be competent above a certain threshold, but we do not have to be more of an autonomous person in order to be entitled to make use of our rights. So, in relation to the right of "self-determination", on grounds of its functional purpose, the concept of autonomy designates a range property (Wikler 1983, 87; cf. Rawls 1971, 508) and is *binary*—either a person is entitled to act on her behalf, or she is not.[10] Autonomous actions in this sense (autonomy$_r$) thus cannot "be autonomous to a different degree" (Quante 2017, 139). The ontic status of being considered a valid decision-making body in one's own affairs is an egalitarian notion. Everyone who is ascribed this status has it equally. Otherwise—if autonomy$_r$ were not an all-or-nothing characteristic—the commitment to moral equality would become problematic, and the fundamental assumption of our legal systems (and of our conceptions of moral rights as well) that, in general, individuals have normative competence for their decisions would lose its foundation and would refer to paternalistic tutelage of the average citizen by members of society endowed with exceptional autonomy.

Behind the functional reason, there is also a normative one for this. In order to achieve normative inclusion and equality, the ontic status of autonomy$_r$—having rights to self-determination and the authority to use them—must include at least most adults. Ascribing rights to persons (whether liberty rights or rights to democratic participation) has to be an extremely inclusive concept. In this perspective, autonomy$_r$ has to define a default position. It is the very sense of ascribing rights within a liberal society based on rights (or in a notion of morality based on equal respect) for this to be as general a concept as possible. Otherwise, it would be impossible to treat persons "as equals" or "with equal concern and respect", as

[9] Of course, some authors in the debate about autonomy$_i$ see this point clearly, e.g. Christman 2015, Sub 1.1., and Beauchamp. 2005, 319 (We need "a way to ensure that ordinary choices qualify as autonomous even when persons have not reflected on their preferences at a higher level and even when they are hesitant to identify with one type of desire rather than another").

[10] It is only through such a low threshold concept of autonomy that the fundamentally *egalitarian*, as well as the *inclusive* character of the concept (or regime) of autonomy can be ensured. It is not until this is accomplished that it makes sense to think about *autonomy-enabling policies* in order to address Joel Anderson's critique that the focus on low threshold conditions fails to protect less-competent groups in society because "the central fact about individual autonomy is how limited the competence of many individuals is and how vulnerable groups are significantly disadvantaged by arrangements in which benefits are distributed in part on the basis of the autonomy-competence that individuals develop 'naturally'" (Anderson 2004).

Ronald Dworkin puts it (Dworkin 1977, 181 et seq., 273–292).[11] This is the main reason why the kind of 'autonomy' referred to here has to be a thin and binary concept. First, as basic competence is a status designator (Christman 2015, Sub 1.1.) and judgments about it have a normative gatekeeping function (Beauchamp and Childress 2013, 114) by distinguishing persons whose decisions should be accepted from those whose decisions should not be accepted, the threshold applied must not be set too high. Second, the number of possible reasons for assuming that a generally competent person is not acting autonomously in the sense of not voluntarily (i.e. not in a way that allows attribution of responsibility) is restricted to the two forms of a lack of voluntariness: coercion, on the one hand, and deceit and error, on the other, the first two being modes of external control. Voluntariness, too, is a binary concept (Wertheimer 1987).

'Thick' concepts of autonomy are generally inadequate and dysfunctional in this regard. Autonomy understood as an ideal and gradual notion and not as an all-or-nothing characteristic is an inherently unequal concept. So when it comes to respecting claims to autonomy as self-determination, e.g. in biomedical ethics or medical law, the question is not whether referring to 'thinner' conceptions of autonomy might suffice. The question is whether any 'thick' concept of autonomy can do the job at all. The answer is clearly negative.

## 8.5 Interrelations and Disruptions

There are positive evaluative interrelations, but also tensions between different 'thick' concepts of autonomy and the 'thin' concept of autonomy as right. (a) In short, the ideal of being one's own person, living one's life according to reasons and motives that are one's own, is a basic moral and political value and might be the very reason why we attribute rights to self-determination in the first place. Vice versa, having rights and being able to claim them is necessary for self-respect and gives a sense to the notion of personal dignity, both of which are prerequisites for leading an autonomous life (Feinberg 1970, 252).[12] As a political ideal, citizens' $\text{autonomy}_i$ is the main source of legitimacy for just political institutions (Christman 2009, 135) and provides reasons for arguing against institutions that attempt to impose a set of ends and values upon the citizens of a society (Dworkin 1988, 10) instead of respecting their right to live their lives in accordance with their own conception of the good. Having basic cognitive and volitional competence (regarding

[11] The very idea of rights involves a commitment to equality, cf. Waldron 2007, 752.

[12] "Having rights enables us to 'stand up like men', to look others in the eye, and to feel in some fundamental way the equal of anyone [...] To respect a person then, or to think of him as possessed of human dignity, simply is to think of him as a potential maker of claims". Self-respect (together with self-trust and self-esteem) serves as a necessary element of several thicker conceptions of $\text{autonomy}_i$ as well, cf. Honneth and Anderson 2005, 132–138; Mackenzie 2008, 525.

rationality, self-control, and the absence of certain mental pathologies) is a prerequisite for both autonomy$_i$ and autonomy$_r$.

(b) However, "personal autonomy" and rights to self-determination are independent concepts with different and conflicting normative functions. The very form of protecting autonomy by granting rights to self-determination must produce heavy tensions between acts which are protected by these rights and the overall goal of realizing 'thick' concepts of autonomy. Rights to self-determination must include the right to act in a way that misses the point or even endangers 'thick' ideals of autonomy. A right to self-determination protects a domain of choice for a person whose reasons for her behavior are necessarily linked in each case to her current self-understanding (Williams 1981, 13). If the ideal of 'thick' autonomy were generally "one of those values for which freedom can be sacrificed" (Oshana 2006a, 126), this would reduce each person as a whole to the role of a mere trustee of her future manifestations of autonomy$_i$ in a way that would be utterly incompatible with the very idea of having rights to self-determination here and now (autonomy$_r$). Such a strategy would disengage a reified concept of "autonomy$_i$" from its bearers and turn it against them.

This is the reason why, in general, no moral or legal consequences follow from the verdict that a sufficiently competent bearer of an autonomy right has not acted "autonomously enough", as measured by 'thick' standards. For this reason, we can conclude that, as far as persons (following Rawls) are self-authenticating sources of valid claims, it is not, as Christman claims, the autonomy$_i$ of the person "that authenticates the validity of these claims" (Christman 2009, 135). If the presumption is "that autonomy confers [...] the authority to make decisions of practical importance for one's life, for one's own reasons, whatever those reasons might be", and "[a]utonomous persons are presumed to have the capacity, the right and the responsibility to exercise this authority" (Mackenzie 2008, 512), then no conception of autonomy$_i$—regardless of whether it is a procedural (content-neutral) or a substantive one (Mackenzie and Stoljar 2000b, 13 et seq.)—qualifies as an adequate criterion for this function.[13] Autonomy$_i$ cannot be a necessary precondition for allowing someone to make use of a right to self-determination, and the very reason for this is that it would indeed be "a mistake to think of personal autonomy$_{[i]}$ as an all or nothing affair and to draw a sharp distinction between autonomous and non-autonomous agents" (Mackenzie 2008, 523).

[13] Mackenzie sees that herself, in part, cf. Mackenzie 2008, 523 ("In the case of citizens' rights to *de jure* political autonomy, the threshold level of competence required ought to be minimal. Agents who meet this minimal level of competence ought to be treated as politically autonomous and entitled to enjoy the rights and liberties that it guarantees, including freedom from the unwarranted paternalistic intervention of the state. To characterize an agent as personally autonomous, however, involves attributing to her capacities that go well beyond this minimal threshold"). Mackenzie's whole argument, however, seems to imply that in moral (as opposed to legal) theory, persons who are not autonomous in a 'thick' sense should *not* have "the capacity, the right and the responsibility to exercise [...] the authority to make decisions of practical importance to one's life, for one's own reasons, whatever those reasons might be" (512).

We face this problem with every ideal-type, (at least moderately) perfectionist notion of personal autonomy, even if it follows a *procedural* account, i.e. is neutral towards the content of a person's values, beliefs, and desires as long as they are endorsed autonomously. What if my upbringing left me with a neurosis that I, upon historically sensitive, adequate self-reflection, am neither willing nor able to endorse nor to identify with, but rather from that I am alienated? Am I allowed to act upon it, nevertheless (although it may not be advisable)? In any case, it is my neurosis, not yours. Am I allowed to choose a partner although my therapist tells me that I am acting upon my unconscious Freudian repetition compulsion? And if I marry her or him anyway, can this person demand me to stick to my valid commitments, i.e. to my marriage contract? Should I be allowed to follow a career plan although I still feel somewhat alienated from the basic values and commitments I am acting upon? The answer, of course, is yes. In other words: interpersonal respect for the autonomy$_r$ of a bearer of rights must not require her to positively identify with or not to be alienated from the trait that motivates her to act. Even people feeling deeply alienated from a personal characteristic have to be allowed to decide how to live their lives, given the persons they are at the moment, even if they are acting out this very characteristic. There may be a right to make alienated decisions as a subform of the general "right to do wrong", as Jeremy Waldron analyzed some 35 years ago (Waldron 1981). In general, a feeling of alienation does not necessarily undermine a person's competence or her ability to act voluntarily. Even neurotic motives and mildly compulsive behavior do not necessarily undercut these features (Feinberg 1986, 168). The same, again, is true for a lack of authenticity, as long as the term "refers to the obligation to live up to one's 'true' self, […] as a form of integrity" (Feinberg 1986, 134; cf. Quante 2017, 129). Even if it comes to decisions of existential importance, we cannot require the bearer of a right to self-determination to reveal some kernel of his true or authentic self. Having a right means not having to give reasons of this kind (Habermas 1996, 119), and inauthentic behavior in general may justify queries, but not interference with people displaying basic competence (which again, for reasons of inclusion, has to be a rather low threshold concept).[14] In the final analysis, the biographical dimension which must be so important in models of personal autonomy$_i$, is widely irrelevant for autonomy$_r$. Therefore, authenticity conditions can only play a very limited role in the concept of autonomy as right to self-determination.

As far as I have a right to self-determination, I have the moral or legal right to make critical life decisions although I am a conformist bore, and I am entitled to act "out of character", to change my life spontaneously in an existentialist manner, discarding biographical consistency, coherence, and rational life plans. In other words: I am allowed to be a bad ('thick') autonomy achiever. If, in one of my existentialist moods, I quit my job, sell my house, and leave my partner voluntarily, but in a manner that rejects my biographical narrative so far, my rational life plan, and

[14] In some contexts, the *stability* of a decision might function as a place-holder for its voluntariness—something which is much less than authenticity.

the relational nexus of my autonomy, I nevertheless have to take moral (and legal) responsibility for the moral (and legal) consequences of my decisions and acts. And this is because 'thick' concepts of autonomy, on the one hand, and the right to self-determination, on the other are functionally independent concepts with different normative functions and must be clearly distinguished.

It becomes even clearer that $\text{autonomy}_i$ cannot be a necessary precondition for allowing someone to make use of a right to self-determination when one regards *substantive* notions of personal autonomy that place restrictions on the *contents* of agents' value commitments, beliefs, and preferences in order to qualify as autonomous (cf. Mackenzie and Stoljar 2000b, 13 et seq.).

Some persons may deliberately forge lives in which autonomy is largely absent, though they possess the capacity and the freedom to do otherwise. Some people become monks leading a life in total obedience or join law firms. Marina Oshana presents the example of a woman, who, having previously enjoyed a successful career as a physician, has since voluntarily chosen to wear a burqa and to lead a life of utter dependence, out of the earnest belief in the sanctity of this role and/or in unquestioned adherence to a religious tradition. Oshana claims that "it is evident that [this] woman is not autonomous" (Oshana 2006a, 104). According to Oshana's specific 'thick' concept, this may be the case.[15] But what follows from this statement? Are we entitled to interfere with her choice? Is this a case for incapacitation, for legal tutelage, for coercive re-education, for taking away her children, for declaring her contracts null and void? Or is it at least a reason to complain that the law will unfortunately not allow us to act in this way, although moral reasons and an adequate theory of 'autonomy' would be clearly in favor of doing so?

Some authors claim that we should not wrongly attribute autonomy to those whose restricted socialization and oppressive life conditions pressure them into internalizing oppressive values and norms (cf. Oshana 1998; id. 2006a. 104; Mackenzie and Stoljar 2000b. See also Oshana 2014). If we agree for the sake of the argument, the question must arise of whether such "$\text{non-autonomous}_i$" people shall be allowed to make their own decisions although their capacity for ideal autonomy has been impaired by their oppressive social environments. Again, the answer, in general, must be yes because making use of individual autonomy rights is very often the only exit option from such environments, whereas denying such people the right to make their own decisions would add insult, degradation, and exclusion to oppression. So if, e.g. according to Natalie Stoljar, "the feminist intuition [...] claims that preferences influenced by oppressive norms of femininity cannot be autonomous" (Stoljar. 2000. 95),[16] taking this notion of $\text{autonomy}_i$ to withhold $\text{autonomy}_r$, i.e. rights of self-determination, from these women would not only amount to quite extensive forms of unwarranted paternalistic interference (Christman. 2004. 157) and to denying existing opportunities for choice, but would also imply that other

[15] Although this is highly questionable. "It is one thing to publically criticize modes of social practice that denigrate their participants, but it is another to define autonomy in a way to claim that those participants are not fully functioning agents at all" (Christman 2004, 158).

[16] See Meyers 2004, 3–12, though.

persons may legitimately serve as decision-makers in these cases. It would amount to specifying a huge (maybe even a majority) group of second-class citizens in need of legal guardians, thus undermining the ontic status of basic equality of persons.[17] If, however, we sever the justificatory ties between such conceptions of autonomy$_{i}$, on the one hand, and respect for autonomy$_{r}$, on the other (which must clearly be done), the claim that we should not wrongly attribute autonomy to those who have internalized oppressive values and norms loses most of its relevance.

(c) The potential dysfunctionality of 'thick' concepts of personal autonomy in certain—but not all—contexts of biomedical ethics can be further elaborated with a look at Michael Quante's text "In Defence of Personal Autonomy" (Quante 2011. See also Quante 2017, 131–150). Against Tom L. Beauchamp's arguments in favor of the conclusion that, in biomedical ethics, we should not refer to personal autonomy (which qualifies the structure of a person's life), but exclusively to action-autonomy (a conception of autonomy$_{r}$) when we use the principle of respect for autonomy in our ethical thinking, Quante argues that introducing a fine-grained conception of the principle of autonomy referring to both action-autonomy and personal autonomy might be an improvement in principlism, the basic idea being "that a person's autonomy can express [it]self both in action-autonomy and in personal autonomy" (Quante 2011, 597).

Quante tries to rebut the thesis that any attempt to draw on personal autonomy as an extension of the principle of respect for autonomy leads to ethically unacceptable consequences in the context of biomedical ethics. And he is certainly right, as "biomedical ethics" deal with a lot of things, including questions of human flourishing and of the good life. There are problems in biomedical ethics which obviously touch the dimension of personal autonomy used to qualify the structure of a person's life or her personal integrity, e.g. long-term care, psychiatry, neurocognitive enhancement, or medical drugs, which have effects on the patient's personality (cf. Quante 2007, 209). So Quante's claim that "a principle of respect for autonomy that is of use to biomedical ethics cannot manage without recourse to autonomy of agency, but must also refer to personal autonomy or the integrity of the personality" (Quante 2017, 132) is certainly true. The question is how the division of labor between autonomy of agency (autonomy$_{r}$) and personal autonomy (autonomy$_{i}$) is conceived.

There seem to be only two options. Concepts of personal autonomy, including Quante's approach, which try to play on the field of action autonomy (or of autonomy as right, as we preferably call it) either address questions of competence (which is the basis for both concepts of autonomy$_{r/i}$), in which case they are relatively trivial, or they really conflate autonomy$_{i}$ as an ideal, gradual, and hence at least

[17] The justified claim that respect for agents whose autonomy is impaired would, as a matter of social justice, entail positive obligations of social institutions to promote the autonomy of these citizens by fostering the social conditions for autonomy (Mackenzie 2008; Honneth and Anderson 2005) would not change anything regarding the two class-system of persons that is created until full justice or recognition in this sense is achieved. Mackenzie's approach does not overcome the correlation of protection and incapacitation that is typical of substantive notions of personal autonomy.

moderately perfectionist notion, and autonomy$_r$. In the latter case, we should expect their demands to prove inadequate or dysfunctional. Michael Quante's approach seems to oscillate between these two possibilities. At least in some refined sense, he claims that "personal autonomy is a necessary condition of autonomy" (Quante 2011, 598) (meaning respect for autonomy, i.e. autonomy$_r$ in the latter case). His example is that consent to become a living organ donor given by a person who is completely incapable of critically reflecting upon her first-order attitude, which was induced in her heteronomously through socialization without ever having been made explicit or endorsed by herself, does not deserve respect. If we take this description seriously, such a choice does indeed not deserve respect because, by all meaningful definitions, this person is not competent to consent. Insofar, and only insofar it refers to basic competence, Quante's thesis is convincing that "in biomedical ethics the respect paid factually to autonomy not only refers to autonomy of agency, but also and always to personal autonomy" (Quante 2017, 140). Referring to *basic* cognitive and volitional competence (regarding rationality, self-control, and the absence of certain mental pathologies), the capacities on which the concept of autonomy$_r$ (autonomy of agency) draws are indeed not independent of the capacities that constitute personal autonomy (autonomy$_i$) (Quante 2017, 142). In short: the concepts of personal autonomy (autonomy$_i$) and autonomy of agency (autonomy$_r$) overlap only insofar as being a "personality with the constitutive capacity of acting autonomously" (Quante 2017, 149) belongs to an adequate threshold definition of basic competence. Quante, however, will not want to entertain a conception of autonomy$_i$ that demands so little. On the other hand, if Quante were to say that the fact in itself that a person is acting upon inexplicit, unreflected motives internalized in her upbringing—or that, if asked, she would not be effectually able to reflect critically upon her first-order preferences, desires, and wishes (Quante 2011, 598)—is sufficient to deny her to make use of her rights (and demand respect in this regard), this would seem to be just another example of the liberty-limiting consequences of the concept of personal autonomy when it is playing on the wrong field.

So there are reasons to assume that, when it comes to "respect for autonomy" or to "respect for persons" guaranteed by individual autonomy rights expressive of one's sovereignty over oneself (autonomy$_r$), as e.g. in the concept of informed consent, the concept of personal autonomy remains misleading and a latent threat to the concept of autonomy$_r$. Quante's remark that "action autonomy [...] and personal autonomy can come in degrees" (Quante 2011, 599) demonstrates that he cannot, or will not, in the final analysis, conceive autonomy$_r$ as the binary ontic status of being a person who can (or cannot) claim a right to self-determination.

Quante concludes that action-autonomy and personal autonomy often "go hand in hand, but in some situations and in some types of case both can diverge (this is why these cases are so puzzling)" (Quante 2011, 599). The answer is that both only go hand in hand as long as they refer to their common basic element, which is competence. In other cases, they have to diverge because they have very different functions within different normative settings, and there is nothing puzzling about that.

## 8.6 The Form of Autonomy Rights

The reason for distinguishing autonomy$_i$ from autonomy$_r$ is not primarily that autonomy also functions as a *political* concept, as "the status marker of an independent citizen whose perspective and value orientation get a hearing in the democratic processes that constitute legitimate social policy" (Christman 2004, 156 et seq.; id. 2009, 219–244). The first reason is the inadequacy of all *moral* concepts of autonomy that cannot account for the respect claimed by autonomous agents, their claim for acknowledgement of their equal moral right to hold views, to make choices, and to take actions based on their values and beliefs.

Of course, there is some awareness for the difference between autonomy$_i$ and autonomy$_r$ in the autonomy debate. Joel Feinberg has analysed four different meanings of "autonomy" in moral and legal philosophy, among them a personal ideal, on the one hand, and a set of rights expressive of one's sovereignty over oneself, on the other. John Christman stresses that "we must keep separate the idea of basic autonomy, the minimal status of being responsible, independent and able to speak for oneself, from ideal autonomy, an achievement that serves as a goal to which we might aspire and according to which a person is maximally authentic and free of manipulative, self-distorting influences. Any plausible conceptualization of basic autonomy must, among other things, imply that most adults who are not suffering from debilitating pathologies or are under oppressive and constricting conditions will be autonomous" (Christman 2015, Sub 1.1.). And as already discussed, Michael Quante, Tom Beauchamp, and others divide the principle of respect for autonomy into two sub-principles: personal autonomy and action-autonomy. The notion of 'action autonomy', however, is too weak and too fuzzy to explain the difference we are looking for (especially as long as we follow the premise that both "action autonomy [...] and personal autonomy can come in degrees" (Quante 2011, 599).

At a closer look, only a certain *form* of protecting autonomy, i.e. protecting autonomy by granting (moral or legal) *rights* to self-determination, can explain some of our most important normative institutions and social practices. The reason for this is the normative structure of rights as specialized normative devices (Sumner 2000, 288, 297), i.e. the distinctive kind of normative work that rights are best equipped to do: guaranteeing "protected options to act" (Kamm 2004, 476) by conferring claims (with corresponding duties for other persons), liberties (with corresponding duties for other persons not to prevent the right-holder from acting within these liberties), and normative powers to individuals. A right is a legally (or morally) "respected choice" (Hart 1982, 189 et seq.). For this task, there is no functional alternative to individual rights. Rights to self-determination and personal liberties are not only "preconditions for self-determination" (Mackenzie 2014), but *its main form of realization*. People become agents of their lives by making choices that are protected and respected.

In light of our practices, rights to self-determination seem to cover a lot of ground, although they do not occupy the whole moral landscape and certainly do not cover all the dimensions of autonomy and the evaluative power of the notion of autonomy. Two final examples have to suffice. The requirement for informed consent and the notion of consent in general can only be justified by the principle of respect for autonomy if autonomy is conceived as a *right* (the bearer of the right, due to a certain normative power conferred by his right, being able to abrogate the corresponding duty of another person not to impair the bodily or personal integrity of the bearer of the right). A right of this sort does not come "in degrees". At the same time, autonomy$_r$ is the main source of our obligations. Similar to the notion of consent, the notions of promising and of contract—the possibility of binding oneself and/or another person, thus changing the nexus of corresponding duties and enhancing and limiting 'action autonomy' at the same time—can also only be explained by the concept of (making use of) a right to self-determination (in the form of a normative power). Again, a right of this sort does not come "in degrees". Consequently, the normative problems dealing with the fact that persons exist through time, and that certain limits on autonomous self-binding for the sake of future autonomy are thus required, can only be grasped and analyzed by distinguishing between autonomy$_r$ (including the right to bind oneself voluntarily, here and now, for the future) and autonomy$_i$ (the value of being one's own person and living one's life as a narrative unity according to reasons and motives that are one's own, at every point in time).

It is the form and intricate anatomy of individual liberty rights (which, in general, do not require any specific content for the choices that the bearer of the right is allowed to make within her right) that calls for the very structure of autonomy$_r$, and vice versa. So the difference between autonomy$_r$ and autonomy$_i$ is not one between basic and ideal autonomy (Christman 2009, Sub 1.1.),[18] it is not a distinction between "metaphysically autonomous" persons and "morally autonomous persons" and not about "relaxing" the standards of higher-order reflection (Beauchamp 2005, 320, 325) until they are low enough to allow for widespread autnomy$_{r.}$ Neither can it be sufficient in cases of conflict between autonomy$_r$ and autonomy$_{i,}$ to assume that the person opting for over-ruling the former in terms of the latter has the burden of proof (Quante 2011, 599). It is rather that we must clearly differentiate between (a) "personal autonomy" (autonomy$_i$), designating a family of ideal, gradual, and hence at least moderately perfectionist notions, on the one hand, and (b) the protection of individual decisions and actions by upholding of rights to self-determination or "authority" (autonomy$_r$). This means that all the quantitative language about one concept of autonomy that comes in "thinner" or "thicker" forms, in a "minimum" or a "full" meaning, in a "basic" or in an "ideal", in a "downgraded" or a "comprehensive" version, is misleading. It seems especially misleading to suggest that, in order

[18] In the final analysis the difference between the mildly perfectionist authenticity criterion e.g. Christman (2004, 2009) suggests on the one hand, and the strong perfectionist view of human values (i.e, the view that values and moral principles can be valid for a person independent of her judgment of those values and principles) that is imported into the account of autonomy by some relational concepts of autonomy on the other hand (see Christman 2004, 146) is also not crucial in this regard. Both conceptions see autonomy as a matter of degree and do not clearly take into account the normative structure of rights that defines the concept of autonomy$_r$ as an ontic status.

to reach an adequate notion of action autonomy (meaning a concept of what it takes to make use of a sovereignty right), we just have to "weaken" the conditions of our theory of personal autonomy that are "too demanding" (Quante 2011, 598) and make them more "realistic" to get this job done. Instead, we are dealing with two different normative concepts with different functions, and we cannot grasp the one by making the other "thicker" or "thinner", or "stronger" or "weaker", respectively.

For clarity, we will ultimately need different words for divergent concepts. Although the term "autonomy", originally meaning "the having or making of one's own laws", is close to the semantic field of "self-determination" and "sovereignty" (Feinberg 1986, 27, 47 et seq., 52 et seq. "personal sovereignty"), we suggest that "autonomy as (moral or legal) right" should no longer be called "autonomy", but forthrightly the "right to self-determination" or, in accordance with Thomas Hobbes, "authority".[19]

## References

Anderson, Joel. 2004. Regimes of Autonomy. *Ethical Theory and Moral Practice* 17: 355–368.

Beauchamp, Tom L. 2005. Who Deserves Autonomy, and Whose Autonomy Deserves Respect? In *Personal Autonomy: New Essays on Personal Autonomy and Its Role in Contemporary Moal Philosophy*, ed. James Stacey Taylor, 310–329. Cambridge/New York: Cambridge University Press.

Beauchamp, Tom L., and James F. Childress. 2013. *Principles of Biomedical Ethics*. 7th ed. New York: Oxford University Press.

Benn, Stanley L. 1976. Freedom, Autonomy, and the Concept of a Person. *Proceedings of the Aristotelian Society* 86: 109–130.

———. 1988. *A Theory of Freedom*. Cambridge: Cambridge University Press.

Berofsky, Bernard. 1995. *Liberation from Self: A Theory of Personal Autonomy*. New York: Cambridge University Press.

Bratman, Michael E. 1987. *Intention, Plans, and Practical Reason*. Cambridge: Harvard University Press.

———. 2007. Planning Agency, Autonomous Agency. In *Structures of Agency: Essays, id*, 195–221. Oxford/New York: Oxford University Press.

Christman, John. 2004. Relational Autonomy, Liberal Individualism and the Social Constitution of Selves. *Philosophical Studies* 117: 143–164.

———. 2009. *The Politics of Persons: Individual Autonomy and Socio-historical Selves*. Cambridge: Cambridge University Press.

———. 2014. Relational Autonomy and the Social Dynamics of Paternalism. *Ethical Theory and Moral Practice* 17: 369–382.

———. 2015, Autonomy in Moral and Political Philosophy. *The Stanford Encyclopedia of Philosophy*, ed. Edward N. Zalta. https://plato.stanford.edu/archives/spr2015/entries/autonomy-moral/. Accessed 4 Apr 2020.

Darwall, Stephen. 1977. Two Kinds of Respect. *Ethics* 88: 36–49.

Dworkin, Ronald. 1977. *Taking Rights Seriously*. Cambridge: Harvard University Press.

Dworkin, Gerald. 1988. *The Theory and Practice of Autonomy*. Cambridge: Cambridge University Press.

[19] "[T]he right of doing any action is called authority", Hobbes 1651, Ch. XVI

Elster, Jon. 1983. *Sour Grapes: Studies in the Subversion of Rationality*. Cambridge: Cambridge University Press.

Feinberg, Joel. 1970. The Nature and Value of Rights. *The Journal of Value Inquiry* 4: 243–260.

———. 1986. *Harm to Self The Moral Limits of The Criminal Law*. New York: Oxford University Press.

Freud, Sigmund. 1972a. Das Ich und das Es. [1923]. In *Studienausgabe Band III*, 273–330. Frankfurt a.M.: Fischer.

———. 1972b. Neue Folge der Vorlesungen zur Einführung in die Psychoanalyse [1932]. In *Studienausgabe Band I*, 448–608. Frankfurt a.M.: Fischer.

Habermas, Jürgen. 1996. *Between Facts and Norms: Contributions to a Discourse Theory of Law and Democracy*. Cambridge, MA: The MIT Press.

Hart, Herbert L.A. 1982. Legal Rights. In *Essays on Bentham: Studies in Jurisprudence and Political Theory*, 162–193. Oxford: Oxford University Press.

Hobbes, Thomas. 1651. *Leviathan or The Matter, Forme and Power of a Common Wealth Ecclesiasticall and Civil*. London: Andrew Crooke.

Honneth, Axel. 1996. *The Struggle for Recognition: The Moral Grammar of Social Conflict*. Cambridge: The MIT Press.

Honneth, Axel, and Joel Anderson. 2005. Autonomy, Vulnerability, Recognition and Justice. In *Autonomy and the Challenges to Liberalism: New Essays*, ed. John Christman and Joel Anderson, 127–149. New York: Cambridge University Press.

Kamm, Frances M. 2004. Rights. In *The Oxford Handbook of Jurisprudence and Philosophy of Law*, ed. Jules L. Coleman and Scott J. Shapiro, 476–513. Oxford: Oxford University Press.

Mackenzie, Catriona. 2000. Imagining Oneself Otherwise. In *Relational Autonomy: Feminist Perspectives on Autonomy, Agency and the Social Self*, ed. Natalie Stoljar, 124–150. New York: Oxford University Press.

———. 2008. Relational Autonomy, Normative Authority and Perfectionism. *Journal of Social Philosophy* 39: 512–533.

———. 2014. Three Dimensions of Autonomy: A Relational Analysis. In *Autonomy, Oppression and Gender*, ed. Andrea Veltman and Mark Piper, 15–41. Oxford: Oxford University Press.

Mackenzie, Catriona, and Natalie Stoljar. 2000a. *Relational Autonomy: Feminist Perspectives on Autonomy, Agency and the Social Self*. New York: Oxford University Press.

———. 2000b. Introduction: Autonomy Refigured. In *Relational Autonomy: Feminist Perspectives on Autonomy, Agency and the Social Self*, 3–31. New York: Oxford University Press.

Meyers, Diana Tietjens. 1989. *Self, Society and Personal Choice*. New York: Columbia University Press.

———. 2000. Intersectional Identity and the Authentic Self: Opposites Attract! In *Relational Autonomy: Feminist Perspectives on Autonomy, Agency and the Social Self*, ed. Catriona Mackenzie and Natalie Stoljar, 151–180. New York: Oxford University Press.

———. 2004. Personal Autonomy and the Paradox of Feminine Socialization. In *Being Yourself: Essays on Identity, Action and Social Life*, ed. Diana Tietjens Meyers, 3–11. Lanham/Boulder: Rowman and Littlefield.

Mill, John Stuart. 1992. On Liberty [1859]. In *On Liberty and Utilitarianism, with an introduction by Isaiah Berlin*. New York: Alfred A. Knopf.

Oshana, Marina. 1998. Personal Autonomy and Society. *Journal of Social Philosophy* 29: 81–102.

———. 2006a. How Much Should We Value Autonomy. *Social Philosophy and Policy* 20: 99–126.

———. 2006b. *Personal Autonomy in Society*. Hampshire: Ashgate.

———. 2014. *Personal Autonomy and Social Oppression*. London: Routledge.

Quante, Michael. 2007. Autonomy for Real People. In *Intentionality, Deliberation and Autonomy: The Action-Theoretic Basis of Practical Philosophy*, ed. Christoph Lumer and Sandro Nannini, 209–226. Aldershot: Asgate.

———. 2011. In Defence of Personal Autonomy. *Journal of Medical Ethics* 37: 597–600.

———. 2017. *Personal Identity as a Principle of Biomedical Ethics*. Cham: Springer.

Rawls, John. 1971. *A Theory of Justice*. Cambridge: The Belknap Press of Harvard University Press.

———. 1988. The Priority of Right and Ideas of the Good. *Philosophy and Public Affairs* 17: 251–276.
———. 2001. *Justice as Fairness: A Restatement*. Cambridge: Harvard University Press.
Raz, Joseph. 1986. *The Morality of Freedom*. Oxford: Oxford University Press.
Steiner, Hillel. 1994. *An Essay on Rights*. Oxford: Oxford University Press.
Stoljar, Natalie. 2000. Autonomy and the Feminist Intuition. In *Relational Autonomy: Feminist Perspectives on Autonomy, Agency and the Social Self*, ed. Catriona Mackenzie and Natalie Stoljar, 94–111. New York: Oxford University Press.
Sumner, Leonard W. 2000. Rights. In *The Blackwell Guide to Ethical Theory*, ed. Hugh LaFollette, 354–373. Oxford: Wiley-Blackwell.
Taylor, Charles. 1985a. Self-interpreting Animals. In *Philosophical Papers, Vol. 1*, 45–76. Cambridge: Cambridge University Press.
———. 1985b. What's wrong with negative liberty. In *Philosophical Papers, Vol.* 2, 211–229. Cambridge: Cambridge University Press.
Thomson, Judith Jarvis. 1990. *The Realm of Rights*. Cambridge: Harvard University Press.
VanDeVeer, Donald. 1986. *Paternalistic Interventions: The Moral Bounds on Benevolence*. Princeton: Princeton University Press.
von Savigny, Friedrich Carl. 1867. *System of the Modern Roman Law, Vol 1*
Waldron, Jeremy. 1981. A Right to Do Wrong. *Ethics* 92: 21–39.
———. 2007. Rights. In *A Companion to Contemporary Political Philosophy*, ed. Robert E. Goodi, Philip Pettit, and Thomas W. Pogge, 745–754. Oxford: Wiley-Blackwell.
Wellmann, Carl. 1985. *A Theory of Rights*. Oxford: Oxford University Press.
Wertheimer, Alan. 1987. *Coercion*. Princeton: Princeton University Press.
Wikler, Daniel. 1983. Paternalism and the Mildly Retarded. In *Paternalism*, ed. Rolf Sartorius, 83–94. Minneapolis: University of Minnesota Press.
Williams, Bernard. 1981. Persons, Character and Morality. In *Moral Luck*, 1–19. Cambridge: Cambridge University Press.



# Chapter 9
# Respecting Personal Autonomy in Bioethics: Relational Autonomy as a Corrective?

**James F. Childress**

**Abstract** Focusing mainly on respect for autonomy, particularly autonomous choices and actions in bioethical decisions, I examine several complexities of enacting this respect through the case of a fourteen-year-old boy who died after being allowed to refuse a necessary blood transfusion on religious grounds (Jehovah's Witness). I argue that thicker concepts of autonomy, closely connected with relational autonomy, direct our attention to aspects of respect for autonomy that are often neglected or underappreciated in much bioethical theory and practice. In particular, they illuminate the interpretive complexity of respecting autonomous choices by focusing attention on the relational context of individuals' decisions, on respect for individuals' social-cultural beliefs and values, and on the temporality of selves, as expressed in their past consent or future consent as well as in—and sometimes in contradiction to—their present consent or dissent. However, it is important not to convert the illuminating and valuable insights from theories of relational autonomy into necessary conditions of autonomous choices and actions and hence of respect for autonomy.

## 9.1 Crisis of Autonomy and Respect for Autonomy in Bioethics

From its beginnings in the late 1960s and early 1970s, bioethics has stressed respect for the autonomy of patients and participants in research. This is not surprising—after all, bioethics emerged in part in reaction to centuries of medical paternalism and exploitation in research, and it was infected with a strongly individualistic orientation, particularly in the U.S., the site and context of much of the early work in the field.

J. F. Childress (✉)
University of Virginia, Charlottesville, VA, USA
e-mail: Jfc7c@virginia.edu



J. F. Childress, M. Quante (eds.), *Thick (Concepts of) Autonomy*, Philosophical Studies Series 146, https://doi.org/10.1007/978-3-030-80991-1_9

Now, however, autonomy and respect for autonomy are under attack—at least certain conceptions are under siege. Critics charge that proponents of autonomy—and many policies and practices in contemporary medicine, health care, and research that are supposedly based on respect for autonomy—make too much of autonomy, extend autonomy too far, and put too much weight on autonomy over against other ethical principles, such as benefitting the patient or protecting the society.

Critics also contend that much work in bioethics does not adequately characterize and interpret autonomous choices and that it thus distorts the processes of consent and refusal. From this standpoint, many conceptions of autonomous choice and consent/ refusal—perhaps the dominant ones—are seen as

- too individualistic, in that they neglect the social context and relational aspects of autonomy;
- too rationalistic, because they ignore the non-rational and emotional aspects of autonomous choices;
- too legalistic, insofar as proponents devote too much attention to laws, regulations, and institutional rules rather than to social practices;
- too formalistic, in view of the excessive attention paid to consent forms over against the process of consent;
- too thin, a common critique of several of these putative deficiencies.

I will examine some key aspects of the standard thin conception of autonomy and respect for autonomy that have come under attack and then explore what one important thicker conception, that of relational autonomy, might add. I will argue that this thicker conception helpfully identifies several aspects of the development and exercise of personal autonomy that further complicate the practice of respect for autonomy. As illuminating and valuable as these insights are, it is important not to convert them into necessary conditions of autonomous choices and actions and of respect for autonomy.

## 9.2 The Principle of Respect for Autonomy (PRA)

What does it mean to *respect persons' autonomous choices and actions*? This cumbersome formulation is more accurate and more adequate than the abstract formulation "respect for autonomy," and it's what I mean in this chapter when I use the phrase *respect for autonomy.*

What is involved in respecting autonomy, in the sense of autonomous choices and actions? "Respect" is more than an attitude; it involves actions. Some *respectful* actions can be stated <u>negatively</u>: <u>not</u> interfering with or attempting to interfere with the autonomous choices and actions of others, and <u>not</u> subjecting or trying to subject those choices to controlling influences.

Two major types of controlling influence are *manipulation of information* and *coercion*. (Beauchamp and Childress, 2019, Chap. 4) When persuasion fails, these two types of intervention are sometimes used in efforts to control others' actions.

Manipulation of information may occur through non-disclosure or deception, while coercion involves a threat of some kind. These interventions are incompatible with respect for autonomous choices and actions. However, it is not inconsistent to say that we respect another person's autonomous choices and actions by non-interference while, at the same time, we try to persuade that person to act differently. It is not even inconsistent to use modes of influence, such as modest incentives and defaults, which shape action but do not control it. (Thaler and Sunstein 2008).

The first formulation of the PRA is negative. My version slightly modifies one offered by Ruth Faden and Tom Beauchamp (1986): *"it is prima facie wrong to subject or attempt to subject the actions (including the choices) of others to controlling influences."* The modifications include the addition of "prima facie" and "or attempt to subject" and "including the choices." This negative principle is expressed and specified in various concrete rights or duties—for example, the right to consent to or refuse medical treatments and the right to liberty of action.

Neither the PRA nor the several specified rights and duties can properly be viewed as absolute. They are at most *prima facie* binding—that is, they are binding, obligatory, other things being equal, and are sometimes justifiably overridden by other principles. An example is protecting public health in an epidemic of serious communicable disease through forcible quarantine against the autonomous choices and actions of recalcitrant citizens.

The PRA is not only negative. It also has clear positive implications in several contexts. In research, medicine, and health care, for instance—where there are fiduciary relations that involve significant differences in power and knowledge, such as the doctor-patient or researcher-subject relationship—the PRA engenders a positive or affirmative obligation to disclose information and to create the conditions for autonomous choices and actions, for instance, by promoting communication and comprehension. As a result, the PRA is reflected in rules of informed consent and refusal but it is not exhausted by or limited to those rules.

I will explore autonomous choices largely through their expression in consents and refusals. Autonomous choices are often made by autonomous persons, but they may also be made in particular situations by persons who would not be described generally or globally as autonomous persons.

## 9.3 Complexities in Respecting Autonomous Choices: A Difficult Case

Even if we accept the PRA, it is neither easy nor simple to act on it. Far from being a mechanical task, respecting autonomous choices and actions is a difficult interpretive task, involving, for instance, judgments of competence or capacity, communication (disclosure of information, comprehension, and response), and voluntariness. This interpretive task entails attentive listening, imagination, discernment, and the like, and these are particularly important in determining what the patient or research subject is really saying. The following case provides a useful point of reference as we examine a few of the complexities of respecting persons' autonomous choices:

### 9.3.1 Case: Death of 14-Year-Old Jehovah's Witness

On November 28, 2007, Dennis Lindberg, age fourteen, died of the effects of acute lymphocytic leukemia and the treatments he was receiving after he refused, on religious grounds (Jehovah's Witness), a blood transfusion that, according to the physicians in this case, could have saved his life and allowed him to live for a few years. His refusal decision was approved by Superior Court Judge John Meyer, who denied a motion filed by the state of Washington to force Dennis to undergo the blood transfusion.

Lindberg was diagnosed with acute lymphocytic leukemia November 8, 2007, and chemotherapy was started but then was stopped because his red blood cell count dropped too low—a common side effect of chemotherapy. Hence the need for the blood transfusion. Medical reports provided to the judge indicated that, with the transfusion and other treatments, Dennis had a 70 percent chance of surviving the next five years.

This case was complicated by Dennis Lindberg's family circumstances. His biological parents wanted him to receive the transfusion, but they did not have legal custody of their son. The boy's legal guardian at the time of his death was his aunt, Dianna Mincin, with whom he had lived for four years, after his father, now a recovering addict, was jailed for drug possession. (According to some reports, both biological parents had been addicted to methamphetamine.) Ms. Mincin, who is a Jehovah's Witness, supported Dennis's decision to refuse a blood transfusion. Jehovah's Witnesses do not want to die in such cases—therefore, this was not a right-to-die case. Indeed, generally Jehovah's Witnesses accept most medical procedures and treatments, but reject blood transfusions for religious reasons.

Hospital administrators reported this case to the state, which then sought a court order to force the transfusion. Courts in the U.S. recognize the rights of adults to refuse potentially life-saving blood transfusions as well as other treatments on religious grounds, but they generally order blood transfusions when medically indicated for children even against parental objections. In reaching his decision, Judge Meyer heard from Dennis's parents, his aunt, social workers, and doctors. Dennis's doctors reportedly supported his decision. Judge Meyer determined that the eighth-grader was a mature minor, who understood that "he's basically giving himself a death sentence." The judge also said: "I don't think Dennis is trying to commit suicide. This isn't something Dennis just came upon, and he believes with the transfusion he would be unclean and unworthy." Finally, according to observers of the court proceedings, the judge indicated that he didn't "believe Dennis's decision is the result of any coercion. He is mature and understands the consequences of his decision."

Some critics of the judge's decision insisted that a fourteen-year-old boy is not competent to make such a life/death decision. According to one critic, adolescents are both more likely to act in ways that seem heroic and very susceptible to influence and pressure. Moreover, they often change their beliefs as they develop. Other critics wondered whether the teenager was experiencing pressure from his immediate caregiver and religious community. In the crisis, his biological parents came from Idaho, where they lived, to indicate their desire for their son to have the transfusion, and to raise questions about whether their son was unduly influenced by his aunt. The father stated: "My sister has done a good job of raising him for the past four years, but her religious beliefs shouldn't be imposed on my son. I want my son to live."

Dr. Benjamin Wilfond, who directs pediatric bioethics at Children's Hospital in Seattle but was not directly involved in this case, focused on several complexities. Dennis would have needed continuing treatments and, with them, repeated transfusions, but it would have been very difficult to force him to cooperate with the treatments over time. As clinicians try to balance protection of children with respect for their autonomous choices, Wilfond observes, "it's not typical to physically restrain children of that age for medical intervention." Dr. Douglas Diekema, another pediatrician and ethicist at Children's Hospital, echoed similar themes—but neither of them could talk specifically abouzzt the details of the Lindberg case. Caregivers are "nervous" in such cases because fourteen-year-olds can have an "adultlike" decision-making process, even though they often change their mind as they get older. Diekema too noted the difficulty of "effectively treat[ing] a kid when he's not going to cooperate."

> In my mind, if there is a role of the court it would be to test a 14-year-old and see just how intense he is about his decision. My approach would be to push it a little further. If he fights you physically, then I'd respect that. But also, are you willing to tie him down every time he needs a transfusion knowing he'll need treatment for the next three years? You'll have a hard time finding a provider willing to do that.

The natural response, Wilfond noted, is to want to do what is necessary to save the young boy: "But imagine if you heard a story about how this individual was strapped down to be given a transfusion, or tackled as he tried to leave the hospital. At fourteen, if you feel strongly about something, you're going to fight back." In contrast to dealing with very young children, caregivers feel "profoundly conflicted" when adolescents are at the center of such cases.

Dianna Mincin's blog (subsequently deactivated) included this comment a few days before her nephew's death:

> For those reading (about) this journey our family has been on that are not one of Jehovah's Witnesses, we compassionately understand your confusion and, perhaps, even your anger at the decision that Dennis and his family have made....While we empathize with your strong feelings, we ask that you attempt to respect Dennis' fight for what he and his family believe so strongly in.[1]

[1] This case was constructed from the following media accounts: Michels 2007; Black 2007a, b; Ostrom 2007.

### *9.3.2 Steps in Respecting Autonomous Choices*

A first step in respecting persons' autonomous choices is to determine whether they have the capacity to act autonomously. This capacity is often referred to as "competence," and I'll use "competence" and "capacity" interchangeably here, although in the United States "competence" is often used in legal contexts. I am viewing the activity and process of determining capacity/competence in ethical rather than legal terms, but sometimes it will be necessary to obtain a legal determination of competence.

Competence or capacity is task specific. We ask whether people have the capacity to do X, Y, or Z. They may lack the capacity to do X but have the capacity to do Y—for example, they may have the capacity to drive an automobile but not to make complex transfers of property. In the case of Dennis Lindberg, the judge determined that, even though he was only fourteen years old, he was a "mature minor," and that he had the capacity to refuse treatments that could prolong his life for perhaps five years (even though, legally, he lacked the competence to obtain a license to drive an automobile). Commentators note that fourteen year olds can have an "adultlike" decision-making process.

Suppose a person lacks competence to give valid consent at a particular time. It is sometimes possible through various interventions to build up or restore a person's capacity for informed consent/refusal. For adults, in contrast to a fourteen-year-old making a life/death decision, we proceed from a presumption of competence and then determine when to disqualify him or her on grounds of limited capacity to make such decisions. Here the fourteen-year-old was presumed to be incompetent, and he had to be evaluated by health care professionals and then by a judge to determine whether he was sufficiently competent to refuse treatment. In practice, questions rarely arise about an adult patient's capacity to decide unless he or she *disagrees* with what the clinician proposes. Probing an individual's capacity to decide or his/her understanding and reasons for decisions in routine health care would be unnecessary, time-consuming, and very costly, apart from a conviction the decision in question is objectively unreasonable or irrational. (Maclean 2009, 248) By contrast, closer attention to evidence about the adult's level of capacity for autonomous choice is warranted when the diagnostic or therapeutic procedures are more invasive or risky.

For a decision to be autonomous the agent needs an adequate understanding of his or her situation, the available options, the probable consequences of different decisions, and so forth. The judge in the Jehovah's Witness case determined that the teenager understood the implications of his decision to refuse a blood transfusion—that he was "basically giving himself a death sentence" through acting on his beliefs. However, some critics observe that fourteen-year-olds often view themselves as heroic and, furthermore, often change their minds about some of their earlier firm convictions as they mature.

Next it is necessary to determine whether a patient's choice is voluntary or made under undue or controlling influence. In the case of Dennis Lindberg, questions were raised about the voluntariness of his choice because of concerns that he was under undue influence or even coercion. His legal guardian was his aunt, a Jehovah's Witness herself, who in a blog asked for respect for "Dennis's fight for what he and his family believe so strongly in." However, Dennis's biological parents opposed his aunt's imposition of her religious beliefs on their son; the inculcation of those beliefs was probably much more subtle and effective than "imposition" would have been for a teenager, who probably would have resisted "imposition." In any event, the judge did not "believe Dennis' decision [was] the result of any coercion."

Finally, it can be difficult to discern what even clearly competent patients really want. That is, what is the actual content of their choices? Even supposing the Jehovah's Witness teenager was competent, understood his situation and the consequences of his decision, and was acting voluntarily, it still could have been difficult to determine exactly what he wanted in the circumstances as they unfolded. It would have been surprising if he had not been ambivalent. One pediatrician-ethicist recommended pushing the interaction further to test "just how intense he is about his decision," to determine whether he would "fight" it. And this pediatrician-ethicist expressed his hope that the judge had done this sort of probing. It is also important to note that sometimes practitioners of the Jehovah's Witness faith appear to give both health care professionals and judges conflicting signals about what they want. I'll return to this later when I discuss cultural beliefs and values.

## 9.4 Relational Autonomy: A Thicker, Richer Conception

### *9.4.1 Components of Relational Autonomy*

Relational autonomy—also called "autonomy in a relational context," "situated autonomy," "contextual autonomy," and so forth—offers an important corrective to some interpretations of the PRA. It directs attention beyond the immediate decision, "the moment of medical decision making" (Sherwin 1998, 32), to the broader context of relations that shape those decisions. Proponents of "relational autonomy," particularly (but not only) feminist thinkers, have helpfully criticized some widespread interpretations and applications of the PRA. I'll focus on relational autonomy rather than on other thick conceptions of autonomy because of limited space, the wide appeal of relational autonomy in bioethics, and its incorporation of elements of some other thick notions. Even so, this is only a brief sketch, hardly representative of the full range of ideas to be found in various conceptions of relational autonomy, and it will concentrate on feminist rather than communitarian conceptions of relational autonomy. (See, for example, the following: Mackenzie and Stoljar, 2000; Stoljar 2014; Friedman 1997; Donchian 2001; Meyers 1997; Sherwin 1992)

Relational autonomists or relationalists find very problematic the picture of the self that sometimes dominates conceptions of autonomy, understood as self-rule or self-governance: individual, self-made, independent, self-interested, isolated and insulated, and so forth. Of course, not all proponents of thin conceptions of autonomy in bioethics or elsewhere accept all these characteristics—these are at most only tendencies. But relational autonomists offer several criticisms of these tendencies.

Self-rule, self-governance, or self-determination does not mean self-creation. The independence emphasized by the PRA does not or should not deny interdependence and neglect the emergence and expression of the self in relationships. For relationists, individuals' autonomous choices are not given, individualistically achieved, or fixed. Instead, we need to recognize how supportive social conditions foster autonomous action. In the words of Susan Sherwin (1998, 39), "Relational autonomy redefines autonomy as the social project it is, but it does not deny that autonomy ultimately resides in individuals."

In the first instance, we think of the impact of close, intimate, interpersonal relationships, particularly families, in shaping the self in both positive and negative ways. This was certainly evident in the case of the Jehovah's Witness teenager—(a) the impact of his biological parents' drug problems and his father's imprisonment, and (b) the impact of his relationship with his aunt, who had become his legal guardian and provided him with a home. Broader social, religious, cultural, and political contexts may also be important. In this case, the teenager's affiliation with a particular religious community was very significant as was his school environment. Even though health care professionals are part of the relational context, in this particular case we don't know much about those relations.

In some situations, the self in self-rule or self-determination may actually be an oppressed self. Hence, it is important to examine the conditions of constraint and limitation under which many exercise—or try to exercise—their autonomy. Attention to social injustice is crucially important for relational autonomists. Even culture may be oppressive; for example, some feminists argue that decisions for breast augmentation or even for breast reconstruction following mastectomy for cancer are unduly influenced and perhaps even, in a way, coerced by the dominant culture.

Furthermore, in health care, medicine, and research, patients and participants/subjects exercise their choices in relation to and with some dependence on clinicians, researchers, and other professionals. This is one factor that gives rise to the positive obligations of respect for autonomy that I mentioned. Through some of these relations, it may be possible to engender, maintain, or restore autonomous choices.

Several themes featured in relational autonomy now appear in more or less standard accounts of respect for autonomy, in part as a result of the extensive and powerful depictions and defenses of relational autonomy in the literature. In the Jehovah's Witness case, a relational approach would have considered carefully the overall relational context—though perhaps no more carefully than the physicians and judge did. Even under a thin account of autonomy much of what relationalists emphasize would have been incorporated because the case involved a minor, a fourteen-year-old. The same might not have been true for many interactions with adults.

I have already noted the relational context that shaped Dennis's decision making: parental drug problems, father's imprisonment, home with and legal guardianship under his aunt, a Jehovah's Witness, for four years; religious community and school community; his physicians and other care givers; and his biological parents who may have arrived on the scene too late to make a difference in view of how rapidly the crisis developed. The relational context also included the judge who probed the teenagers' views. As previously noted, one pediatrician-ethicist indicated that the role of the court should have been to determine the *intensity* of Dennis's beliefs—"to push back a little further" to determine whether he "fights you." Since the treatment over time would have required repeated transfusions, there would have been on-going fights, and health professionals opposed using physical force in order to provide the rejected blood transfusion.

In sum, valuable insights and helpful correctives to common understandings and misunderstandings of the PRA have emerged from conceptions of "relational autonomy." Some of these correctives were already implicit in or have since been incorporated into the standard approach. No doubt, virtually any thin approach would attend to relational autonomy in the care of minors, but proponents of relational autonomy contend that it should extend to all throughout health care. However, not all approaches to or implications and applications of relational autonomy—and there are many different conceptions—are defensible.

### 9.4.2 *Relationally Responsible Choices: A Necessary Condition of Autonomy?*

One conception of "relational autonomy" is problematic because it builds a notion of relational, moral responsibility into the conception of autonomy itself. Some interpreters hold that a relationally autonomous choice is one that recognizes its societal repercussions and decides and acts accordingly.[2] Similar issues are raised by "principled autonomy," which Onora O'Neill (2002, 2003) and others, following Kant, use to build a notion of responsibility into autonomy (hence, "principled autonomy.") (See also Manson and O'Neill 2007) From this standpoint, we are not choosing autonomously if we do not attend to the impact of our actions on others.[3]

My approach is quite different, as developed in *Principles of Biomedical Ethics* co-authored with Tom Beauchamp: people's autonomous choices may be unethical in failing to attend to relational responsibilities and to negative impacts on others; hence, these autonomous choices may sometimes be justifiably overridden. That these choices are unethical does not disqualify them as autonomous; it only means that they are not ethically justifiable all things considered. And since, like other

[2] See the depiction of relational autonomy in McLean 2010.

[3] It is unclear whether and to what extent the Jehovah's Witness teenager considered the impact of his refusal of the blood transfusion on others.

ethical principles (in the Beauchamp-Childress framework), the PRA is only *prima facie* binding, it too can be justifiably overridden under some circumstances. Take, for instance, a refusal to follow an order of quarantine in a public health crisis. That refusal could be an autonomous choice but justifiably overridden to protect others.

### 9.4.3 Respect for an Individual's Social-Cultural Beliefs and Values

Relationalists also stress the larger social-cultural context that shapes individuals' choices, sometimes to the extent of practically constituting their identities, not merely functioning as a causal background. Of course, bioethics needs to attend to various and significant social-cultural contexts of choices. This is crucially important in multicultural societies. How we should do this requires careful thought.

Several empirical studies challenge what they take to be the dominant Western bioethical view of respect for patient autonomy and its implications for determining how much patients should know and decide. All in all, these studies enrich our understanding of the PRA and its applications, but their findings require careful interpretation, both theoretically and practically.

In one study, researchers in California studied the differences in the attitudes of elderly subjects (65 years or older) from four different ethnic backgrounds (Korean American, Mexican American, European American, and African American) toward the roles the individual patient and the family should play in the disclosure of a diagnosis and prognosis of a terminal illness, such as cancer, and in decision making at the end of life. The study enrolled 800 subjects, 200 from each of the four ethnic groups. Following is the researchers' summary of their main findings:

> Korean Americans (47%) and Mexican Americans (65%) were significantly less likely than European Americans (87%) and African Americans (88%) to believe that a patient should be told the diagnosis of metastatic cancer. Korean Americans (35%) and Mexican Americans (48%) were less likely than African Americans (63%) and European Americans (69%) to believe that a patient should be told of a terminal prognosis and less likely to believe that the patient should make decisions about the use of life-supporting technology (28% and 41% vs 60% and 65%). Instead, Korean Americans and Mexican Americans tended to believe that the family should make decisions about the use of life support. (Blackhall et al. 1995, 820–825).

This study determined that the attitudes toward disclosure and toward decision making primarily correlated with ethnicity and secondarily with respondents' years of education and personal experiences of illness and medical decision making.

The researchers indicate that their study shows that the "belief in the ideal of patient autonomy is far from universal." (Blackhall et al. 1995, 824) They contrast that ideal with a "family-centered model," which emphasizes the individual's web of relationships, and tends to place a higher value on "the harmonious functioning of the family than on the autonomy of its individual members." (Blackhall et al.

1995, 825) Hence, there are two divergent models of medical decision making: a family-centered model and a patient-centered model.[4]

The researchers recommend that physicians "ask their patients if they wish to receive information and make decisions or if they prefer that their families handle such matters." (Blackhall et al. 1995, 820) That recommendation is a way both to *recognize* and to *respect* patients' autonomy. Rather than abandoning the ideal of patient autonomy, as the researchers sometimes suppose, this permits individuals to exercise their autonomy by choosing the model they prefer for disclosure of information and decision-making—a patient-centered or a family-centered one. Even a patient's choice of a family-centered model can be an autonomous choice.

In places the authors seem to admit that we don't have to abandon our commitment to individual autonomy or to (the legal doctrine of) informed consent. Instead, they say (Blackhall et al. 1995, 825), what is required is "*broadening* our view of autonomy so that respect for persons includes respect for the cultural values they bring with them to the decision-making process" (italics added). Generally I concur with this conception of broadening the view of respect for autonomy, in contrast to claims of abandonment—perhaps the researchers' earlier statements should be read as an abandonment of excessively *individualistic* notions of autonomy.[5] However, my concurrence includes a strong cautionary note. It is important to avoid reading *individuals*' values off the *cultural* values they generally affirm, or *individuals'* narratives off their *cultural* narratives.

Each year I teach a broad, comparative course on Religion and Medicine for fourth-year medical students, and I caution the participants as follows: when we learn what a particular religious or cultural tradition affirms, we cannot conclude from this that an individual affiliated with that tradition thinks or believes or acts in a particular way. The individual is not a mere subset of a social-cultural tradition even if that tradition has, in part, shaped the person's identity and the person still identifies with it. We cannot suppose that an observant religious person necessarily holds or acts on a belief or value generally associated with, or even authoritatively promulgated by, his or her particular religion.

This too is important for our central case. It is natural to assume that a self-identified and committed Jehovah's Witness will consistently and adamantly refuse a blood transfusion as contaminating and polluting, based on that tradition's formal statements of beliefs and values. Nevertheless, some Jehovah's Witnesses, perhaps a small minority, actually believe that *consent* to the transfusion, rather than the *transfusion* itself, contaminates the individual—no consent, no contamination! And, according to transcripts of a number of bedside interviews conducted by judges of adult Jehovah's Witnesses who refuse to consent to a blood transfusion recommended by physicians, these patients may appear even to welcome or invite health care professionals and courts to help them through this loophole in their beliefs—for

[4] See also the critique of what the author sees as the individualistic version of respect for autonomy in principlism, from the perspective of Japanese culture, in Traphagan 2013.

[5] See McLean (2010) for a discussion of both individualistic and relational conceptions of autonomy in English law.

some, a court-ordered (but unconsented to) transfusion would not have negative religious repercussions. (Childress 2015) Health care professionals and judges are in a difficult ethical and legal bind when in some circumstances the adult Jehovah's Witness does not want to die but cannot consent to a potentially life-saving blood transfusion without jeopardizing his or her religious standing. Some judges have authorized the transfusions while others have declined to do so. (Childress 2015).

The suggestion above that the Jehovah's Witness teenager's resolve could be tested by seeing whether he would put up a fight should be understood in this connection. As a result of his probing, perhaps the kind required by relational autonomy, the judge understood the teenager to believe that "with the transfusion he would be unclean and unworthy"—even if the court ordered it without his consent or against his refusal. But, as also indicated earlier, we actually don't know what kind of probing the judge used.

In summary, understanding the patient's social-cultural context is very important for clinicians in both disclosing information and interpreting patients' responses. But individuals' appropriations and expressions of their socio-cultural traditions and values may be quite idiosyncratic—they may even reject those traditions and values at some key points relevant to the decision at stake. This holds whether these social-cultural traditions and values function causally, as background conditions, or constitutively for those individuals.

### 9.4.4 Respect for Temporally Extended Selves

Another source of complexity in respecting autonomy stems from the fact that we are "temporally extended selves." (Baumann 2008) We exist in and through time and our choices and actions occur over time. Among the several theorists of relational autonomy who have emphasized this, Susan Sherwin (1998, 35) observes: "Under relational theory, selfhood is seen as an ongoing process rather than as something static or fixed." In discharging our obligations under the PRA, we not only have to determine whether a person is choosing autonomously and what he or she chooses, but we also have to put that person's current consents and dissents in a broad temporal context with attention to the past and the future as well as the present. As temporal beings through and through, we frequently express different views and preferences at different times.

Not surprisingly, respecting autonomy in bioethics often focuses on the present moment—for example, do we have the patient's or prospective research subject's informed consent or refusal at this time? However, respecting persons and their autonomous choices becomes very complex when we consider their temporality: Which choices and actions should we respect? In particular, is it ever justifiable to override a patient's present choices and actions in the light of his or her past or (anticipated) future choices and actions? Most dramatically, which person do we respect?

***Past or Prior Consent*** Past or prior consent/refusal poses no problem if the patient cannot currently autonomously express his or her wishes, perhaps because of mental incapacity. As in the case of advance directives, we respect personal autonomy by acting on that past or prior statement of preference, what is sometimes called precedent autonomy. (Davis 2007) Matters become more problematic, however, when a person's present choices appear to contradict those prior choices. Sometimes the person may have even made those prior choices to prevent future changes.

For example, in one case, a 28-year-old man decided to terminate chronic renal dialysis because of his poor quality of life and the burdens his condition and its treatment created for his family—his medical conditions included diabetes, legal blindness, and progressive neuropathy that rendered him unable to walk. At his request, his wife and physician finally agreed to this arrangement: when he stopped dialysis, he would receive medication to relieve his pain while he died, and he would not be put back on dialysis even if he requested it. While dying in the hospital, the patient awoke complaining of pain and asked to be put back on dialysis. The patient's wife and physician decided to act on the man's earlier request that he be allowed to die, and he died four hours later. (Beauchamp and Childress 2019, 111–112)

In my judgment, the spouse and physician should have put the patient back on dialysis in view of his current request and the irreversibility of acting in accord with his earlier, now repudiated, statements. After putting him back on dialysis, they could have determined whether he had autonomously revoked his prior choice. Suppose he said, "Damn it, I told you not to put me back on dialysis whatever I said…." Then they could have proceeded again with greater confidence.

As this case suggests, it is sometimes critically important to determine whether people have autonomously revoked their previous consents/refusals. In such cases, we need to assess a person's level of autonomy over time in order to determine whether the apparent revocation of previous consents or dissents is autonomous. The PRA requires that we attend to both a person's prior consent/refusal and his or her present revocation when there is a conflict, but the present revocation takes priority if it is autonomous.

An important interpretive perspective in respecting autonomous choices is that of narrative unity, integrity and authenticity. (See Miller 2014) One question that often arises is how a patient's current choices fit in with the choices he or she has made over time and in accord with his or her character. Narrative unity and integrity, for example, involve wholeness and constancy over time.

Authenticity, according to one philosopher, means that "an action is consistent with the attitudes, values, dispositions and life plans of the person." (Miller 2014) Its intuitive idea is "acting in character." Learning whether a person's present choice or action is consistent or inconsistent with that person's life plan and risk budget as embodied over time may help us determine, for example, whether a revocation is genuine. On the one hand, we may wonder whether a person's actions are autonomous if they are out of character (e.g., a person's sudden and unexpected decision to discontinue a needed medical treatment). On the other hand, we are less likely to challenge actions as non-autonomous if they are in character (e.g., a committed Jehovah's Witness's refusal of a blood transfusion).

These ideas of narrative unity, integrity, and authenticity are important, but it would be a mistake to make them criteria for determining whether choices are autonomous. At most, actions apparently out of character and inauthentic raise caution flags that warn others to press for explanations and justifications in order to determine whether those actions are in fact autonomous. However, we cannot rule out in advance the possibility of a change or even a conversion in basic values.

***Future or Deferred Consent*** Suppose a patient refuses a potentially life-sustaining treatment because of pain, suffering, and apparently limited life prospects. In some such situations clinicians may have good reason to believe that if the patient were kept alive by a particular treatment that she is now refusing, she would eventually ratify the coercive or deceptive treatment on her behalf, perhaps even thanking the professional. Such retrospective ratification does occur in some cases.

But the question is whether *anticipated* future ratification justifies—or helps to justify—acting now against a patient's current express choices in order to respect who that person will become rather than who she currently is. I would argue that predicted future ratification is neither necessary nor sufficient to justify paternalistic interventions against current choices. At most, a patient's probable future ratification may provide supporting (but still inconclusive) evidence that the conditions for justified paternalistic interventions have been met. It is also important to note that the intervention may have changed the person in the process.

## 9.5 Conclusions

I have argued that thicker concepts of autonomy, closely connected with relational autonomy, can enable us—and, indeed, have enabled us—to see more clearly aspects of respect for autonomy that have often been neglected or downplayed in much bioethical theory and practice. In the process, they help us understand better the interpretive complexity of the PRA. This complexity is unavoidable because people—the very people whose autonomy we are to respect—are complex, as indicated by conceptions of relational autonomy.

A danger is that these valuable indicators for respecting autonomous choices might be made into necessary conditions for autonomy, conditions that would then ground respect for autonomy. This would set a standard for autonomous actions that is too high and too demanding and would thus deprive ordinary decision-makers of the protection and support needed for their autonomous choices and actions. It could even create the specter of paternalistic interventions in the name of thicker conceptions of autonomy. The worry is that we will be tempted to override a person's specific minimally but sufficiently autonomous choice because it fails to satisfy the standards of thicker conceptions of autonomy.

## References

Baumann, Holger. 2008. Reconsidering Relational Autonomy: Personal Autonomy for Socially Embedded and Temporally Extended Selves. *Analyse & Kritik* 30: 445–468.

Beauchamp, Tom L., and James F. Childress. 2019. *Principles of Biomedical Ethics*. 8th ed. New York: Oxford University Press.

Black, Cherie. 2007a. Boy dies of leukemia after refusing treatment for religious reasons. *Seattle Post-Intelligencer*, November 29

———. 2007b. Jehovah's Witnesses: Boy's death ends battle. *Seattle Post-Intelligencer*, November 29.

Blackhall, Leslie J., Sheila T. Murphy, Gelya Frank, et al. 1995. Ethnicity and Attitudes toward Patient Autonomy. *JAMA: Journal of the American Medical Association* 274: 820–825.

Childress, James F. 2015. Jehovah's Witness Refusal of Blood Transfusions: Ethical and Legal Controversies. Unpublished paper.

Davis, J.K. 2007. Precedent Autonomy, Advance Directives, and End-of-Life Care. In *The Oxford Handbook of Bioethics*, ed. Bonnie Steinbock, 349–374. New York: Oxford University Press.

Donchian, Anne. 2001. Understanding Autonomy Relationally: Toward a Reconfiguration of Bioethical Principles. *Journal of Medicine and Philosophy* 26 (4): 365–386.

Faden, Ruth R., and Tom L. Beauchamp. 1986. *A History and Theory of Informed Consent*. New York: Oxford University Press.

Friedman, Marilyn. 1997. Autonomy and Social Relationships: Rethinking the Feminist Critique. In *Feminists Rethink the Self*, ed. Diana Tietjens Meyers. Boulder: Westview Press.

Maclean, Alasdair. 2009. *Autonomy, Informed Consent and Medical Law: A Relational Challenge*. Cambridge: Cambridge University Press.

Mackenzie, Catriona, and Natalie Stoljar, eds. 2000. *Relational Autonomy: Feminist Perspectives on Autonomy, Agency, and the Social Self*. New York: Oxford University Press.

McLean, Sheila. 2010. *Autonomy, Consent and the Law. Biomedical Law and Ethics Library*. London: Routledge-Cavendish.

Manson, Neil C., and Onora O'Neill. 2007. *Rethinking Informed Consent in Bioethics*. Cambridge: Cambridge University Press.

Meyers, Diana Tietjens, ed. 1997. *Feminists Rethink the Self*. Boulder: Westview Press.

Michels, Scott. 2007. Judge Allowed 14-Year-Old Jehovah's Witness to Refuse Potentially Lifesaving Care Leukemia Patient Dies After Refusing Blood Transfusion for Religious Reasons. *ABC News Internet Ventures*, with reporting from the Associated Press, November 29.

Miller, Bruce. 2014. Autonomy. In *Bioethics [formerly The Encyclopedia of Bioethics]*, ed. Bruce Jennings, 4th ed., 302–307. New York: Macmillan Reference.

O'Neill, Onora. 2002. *Autonomy and Trust in Bioethics*. Cambridge: Cambridge University Press.

———. 2003. Autonomy: The Emperor's New Clothes. *Proceedings of the Aristotelian Society* sup. 77: 1–21.

Ostrom, Carol M. 2007. Mount Vernon leukemia patient, 14, dies after rejecting transfusions, *The Seattle Times*, November 29.

Sherwin, Susan. 1998. A Relational Approach to Autonomy in Health Care. In *The Politics of Women's Health: Exploring Agency and Autonomy*, The Feminist Health Care Ethics Research Network, coordinator Susan Sherwin, 19–47. Philadelphia: Temple University Press.

———. 1992. *No Longer Patient: Feminist Ethics and Health Care*. Philadelphia: Temple University Press.

Stoljar, Natalie. 2014. Feminist Perspectives on Autonomy. *The Stanford Encyclopedia of Philosophy* (Spring 2014 Edition), ed. Edward N. Zalta, URL = http://plato.stanford.edu/archives/spr2014/entries/feminism-autonomy/

Thaler, Richard H., and Cass R. Sunstein. 2008. *Nudge: Improving Decisions About Health, Wealth, and Happiness*. New Haven: Yale University Press.

Traphagan, John. 2013. *Rethinking Autonomy: A Critique of Principlism in Biomedical Ethics*. Albany: State University of New York Press.

# Chapter 10
# Patients' Decision-Making Competence: Discontents with a Risk-Relative Conception

**Bettina Schoene-Seifert**

**Abstract** Regarding patients' valid informed consent to treatment, it is a still contested issue, whether the level of required decisional competency should mirror the riskiness of the treatment at stake. This chapter attempts to refute such a risk-relative conception of competence (RRCC) on the basis of a systematic analysis of relevant arguments, both conceptual and normative ones. A misconception of autonomy's proper value and attribution as well as the danger of a hidden paternalism are among the main objections against RRCC.

## 10.1 Introduction

Informed consent requirements are a cornerstone of modern biomedical ethics and medical law. "Gate-keeping"[1] for the whole procedure of soliciting a patient's personal consent to medical interventions is his or her mental *competence*. Taking competence as existing in degrees, some ethicists have proposed a "sliding-scale" conception of those mental capacities (making up for competence) that are deemed necessary for a patient's valid consent. In a nutshell, the suggestion requires a higher degree of decisional abilities, the higher the (potential) harm of the medical decision at stake. Although ethicist James Drane (1985) is often regarded as the originator of this idea, others made similar suggestions even before him, not the least the legendary President's Commission in 1982.[2] Since then, this suggestion of a

[1]To my best knowledge, the now common *gatekeeping* metaphor was coined by Faden and Beauchamp 1986, p.287ff.

[2]Roth et al. 1977; President's Commission 1982, Vol 1, p.60ff. Similarly: Gaylin 1982. I owe the first reference to Culver and Gert 1990, p.632 and the following ones to Beauchamp 1991, p.70.

B. Schoene-Seifert (✉)
Institute for Medical Ethics, History and Philosophy of Medicine, Münster, Germany
e-mail: bseifert@uni-muenster.de



J. F. Childress, M. Quante (eds.), *Thick (Concepts of) Autonomy*, Philosophical Studies Series 146, https://doi.org/10.1007/978-3-030-80991-1_10

sliding-scale or, as I prefer to call it in line with probably dominant terminology, a *risk-related*[3] conception of competence (RRCC) has been adopted by many clinicians, psychologists, and bioethicists. They welcome it as a reconstruction of common clinical practice and as allowing a "balance between the competing values of self-determination and wellbeing that are to be served by a determination of competence" (Buchanan and Brock 1989, p.64). Others, however, have criticized the risk-related conception for various conceptual and normative reasons, thus arguing for the alternative, i.e. a *fixed* concept of patients' decision-making competence. Notably, although a controversial and high-level exchange of arguments among some bioethicists took place around the 1990s,[4] nothing like an expert consensus or *explicitly* adopted majority view on this practically important issue has yet been achieved.

In this paper I attempt to provide a systematic analysis of relevant arguments, critically reconsidering older ones and elaborating on what I consider some new concerns. As a result, I will join the camp of RRCC-opponents, holding that only a *fixed* concept of decisional competency fits the very reasons why we (should) value autonomy – despite some initial plausibility to the contrary. More specifically, I will argue that not only hidden paternalism in matters of risk-taking, but also a dangerously inflationary attribution of autonomy (e.g. in cases of severe mental disturbance) with a number of problematic implications are lingering in RRCC's background. In any case, I want to show that the RRCC issue still or anew deserves bioethical attention.

## 10.2 Decision-Making Competence: Preliminary Aspects

### *10.2.1 A Precondition for Valid Authorization*

In medico-legal and bioethical contexts 'competence' is a common shortcut for patients' *decisional* competence[5] and as such I will use it, too. The main medical area in which this concept plays a role is the context of informed consent, where

---

[3] There are several important ambiguities in the term 'risk', well-known from other fields of decision-making analysis: (1) risks can be understood and quantified either as the mere likelihood that *some* negative effect might occur, or else as a *joint* parameter (in standard decision theory: the mathematical product) of the probability and quality of possible negative effects. Moreover, risks can be taken (2) as gross or net, (3) subjective or objective, as well as (4) expected *ex ante* or realized *ex post.* For the *principled* purpose of this paper it seems acceptable to understand 'risk' as some non-negligible probability of some non-negligibly *net*-harmful consequences assessed from an intersubjective *ex ante* perspective – and to leave all the detail questions open.

[4] See, for example, the following: Macklin 1987; Buchanan and Brock 1989; Culver and Gert 1990; Beauchamp 1991; Wicclair 1991, 1997; Wilks 1997, 1999; Cale 1999; Checkland 2001; DeMarco 2002.

[5] Some authors insist that competence is a purely legal term: e.g. Ganzini et al. 2004, p.264, but common usage proves to the opposite.

patients are asked to make personalized decisions for or against suggested medical interventions in either clinical or research contexts.[6] For the sake of brevity I will in the following only speak of decision-making on medical 'treatment' options.

Following the dominant understanding, the main impetus of the informed consent doctrine is to grant competent patients decisional *authority* with regard to their medical treatment – i.e. choosing between professionally appropriate interventions or refusing any of them.[7] Ethically, this "autonomous authorization model of informed consent"[8] was pioneered and notably fleshed out more than 30 years ago by US-bioethicists Beauchamp, Childress, and Faden (Beauchamp and Childress [1]1979; Faden and Beauchamp 1986) and has since become the governing model. According to common legal, ethical, and practical standards,[9] a patient's consent should be authoritative or binding, if it fulfils the requirements of originating from a patient who (i) is competent, (ii) actually understands what he is consenting to, and (iii) decides voluntarily. These triple core requirements mirror the leading understanding of valid consent as *autonomous* authorization (AA) given that they correspond to the three standard criteria of autonomous action in general.

Thus, attribution of competence in the context of medical decision-making functions as an entrance ticket that entitles a patient to make *authoritative* self-regarding treatment decisions and to assume responsibility for part of this choice. An important other part of responsibility stays, of course, with caretakers who must properly recommend and explain treatment options and refrain from interfering with voluntary decision-making. But the final authorization rests with the patient. This is not the place for analyzing the underlying reasons various stakeholders have to welcome or deplore this partial shift of responsibility. One can admit of informed consent policies sometimes being motivated by caretakers' fear of legal liability or their wish to personally reduce some of their own responsibility, to shorten patient contact etc. (See O'Neill 2007) However, such secondary motivations do not rule out a serious ethical concern with respecting patients' personal *autonomy*. Despite the enormous variety of different concepts of personal autonomy in ethics that I cannot even start to discuss in this paper, the core idea of patient autonomy in bioethics is

---

[6] I use the term 'intervention' in a loose way, covering therapeutic, diagnostic, and preventive procedures, hospitalizations etc. Other patient decisions requiring competence may regard specific, often controversial interventions *primarily* asked for by patients such as elective abortions, assistance in suicide, or enhancement.

[7] Thus, in terms of *absolute* authority, patients' decisional power is that of a veto power. Whenever there are several reasonable options patients are, moreover, authorized to choose among them. Granting respect for patients' autonomy in this standard sense is clearly distinct from *wish-fulfilling medicine* – in contrast to some common suspicions.

[8] "Autonomous authorization" was identified as the primary function of informed consent by Faden and Beauchamp 1986. It was proposed as a label by Miller and Wertheimer 2011. I cannot here discuss their (and other authors') recent objections to the AA-model for consent to biomedical research.

[9] In the following my focus will be on ethical considerations and literature. However, I certainly acknowledge that relevant debates are taking place in the legal(-ethical) literature, e.g. Alexander 1996; Amelung 1992.

the notion of (optional) authority in personalizing one's medical treatment with an eye also on one's non-medical values and preferences. It is this specific task that must dictate patient competence. As we shall see, it thereby renders RRCC a questionable idea.

Since the early attempts to flesh out ethically sound criteria for valid informed consent, scholars have had, however, to differentiate between ideal and non-ideal approaches, where the latter take into consideration that 'ordinary' people often make decisions under less than optimal conditions (inner and outer ones) and that 'ordinary' medical personnel most often have to judge their patients' decision-making within limited time and with restricted expertise. Clearly, such real-life obstacles to the ideal of fully autonomous consent (whatever that is, exactly) should be remedied to the extent possible. But in addition, informed consent *policies* should, according to the standard view, already accept substantially autonomous decisions as valid. Moreover, policies must make a set of reasonable presumptions and set certain standards of evidence for the validity of consent.[10] One such element is the presumption of competence in the case of most conscious adult patients. In the words of bioethicist Govern den Hartogh's:

> We assume in the case of most patients, and of most persons generally, that they are competent in all their decisions until a reason for doubt arises, we do not investigate their competence in the case of each and every decision. That would be impossible in practice, but there is more fundamental reason for the presumption as well: we can only take each other seriously and treat each other as moral equals on this basis. (Hartogh 2016 p.72; likewise: Buchanan and Brock 1989, p.57ff )

As Hartogh goes on to explain, the most prominent "reason for doubt" regarding patients' competence is that their decisions deviate from their physicians' treatment recommendations. Given that these recommendations are commonly based on professional comparative risk/benefit assessments of available treatment options, a deviation is likely to appear puzzling, unreasonable, or irrational. Thus, this might justify and trigger a process of competence assessment because one of several possible explanations for a judgmental deviance between a physician and her patient is the latter's lack of competence to properly make the judgment and decision at stake. Hence, according to mainstream assumptions, a decision's irrationality is to be taken as an indicator for *potential* incompetence, not as the latter's proof – although the conceptual relation between incompetence and irrationality proves somewhat tricky and controversial (see next paragraph).

[10] According to my understanding, the difference between a given consent's *real* qualities and its assessment by legal and institutional policies corresponds to the difference between what Faden and Beauchamp (1986, p.277f.) have called informed consent (sense1) and (sense2). In any case, the gap between hypothetical ethical requirements for any single case of decision-making and actual policy requirements can account for some puzzling questions. They regard, e.g., issues of self-induced non-understanding, robust false beliefs, or imprudent decision-making by competent patients. In all such cases that I cannot here pursue any further, ethically legitimate policy might accept resulting decisions *as if* sufficiently autonomous and 'informed' although they do not fulfil the standard criteria.

### 10.2.2 A Set of Abilities

Obviously, competence does not consist in one single element but rather in a set of mental capacities. One minimalist account asks for (i) a capacity to understand and communicate[11] and (ii) a capacity to appreciate various treatment alternatives. On closer look, this "understand-and-appreciate account of competence" (Culver and Gert 1990, p.639; likewise, Checkland 2001, p.36) can only serve as a rough shortcut, which I will deliberately use in the following. However, for the purpose of conceptual, ethical, psychological, or clinical analyses both additions and further fine-graining would be necessary.

A patient's appreciation, for instance, presupposes the capability to deliberate, i.e. to process information in a basically consistent way and to be potentially responsive to new aspects and arguments. But it also needs the capability to assess available treatment options in the light of one's personal values and preferences, thus making subjective *comparative* evaluations. Again, a background condition of such evaluations must be what is usually called "the possession of a (stable) set of personal values".[12] This last item cannot properly be called a capability in the strict sense. Rather, as common-sense psychology already suggests, such value set is the result of a person's biographical experiences over time, not the least formed by personal relations, social determinants, and a more or less conscious reflection of who one wants to be. In debates on how to conceptualize autonomy, this "evaluative self-image" (Quante 2011, p.174ff) plays a key role in at least two aspects. One aspect concerns the logical and substantial links between the focal autonomy of a patient's treatment decision and her personal autonomy on a more global scale. The other aspect concerns the ways in which the acquisition of one's value-set can be disturbed in autonomy-violating ways (e.g. by repression, traumatization, or brainwashing). Both aspects can be disregarded in the context of the sliding scales dispute that mainly focuses on patients' *cognitive* sophistication or deficits.

Cognitive competence, too, is an issue of on-going interdisciplinary discussion among legal and philosophical scholars as well as among cognitive scientists. Debates concern its composite nature, its interdependence with emotional or volitional capacities, and its practical assessment in bedside situations.[13] All of this will

[11] Communication of choice is sometimes listed as a necessary element of competence. Strictly speaking, this is not required for decision-making as such, but rather for its operationalization (think of a locked-in patient who might well come to a decision but might under unfortunate circumstances not be able to communicate it). However, in *practically* oriented lists communication is a standard item. Moreover, communication usually has an important role in the process of patient understanding.

[12] Hence, various authors add "the possession of a set of values and goals" as a third minimalist requirement. Compare Wicclair 1991, p.91; Buchanan and Brock 1989, p.23.

[13] To quote Louis Charland, bioethicist and philosopher of cognitive sciences: "The combined theoretical and practical nature of decisional capacity in the area of consent is probably one of the things that makes it so intellectually compelling to philosophers who write about it. But this is still largely uncultivated philosophical territory. One reason is the highly interdisciplinary and rapidly

again be ignored in the following – in favour of a somewhat sketchy understand-and-appreciate concept of competence. Whatever its more precise nature, its realization surely is a gradual, not a binary phenomenon. People can memorize, understand, deliberate, appraise, or make a choice with gradual goodness.[14] (Charland 2015, sec. 1) Against this background it is commonly and reasonably agreed, that an authoritative patient decision only needs a sufficient amount of each of the capabilities that are constitutive of competence, thus resulting in a *sufficient* degree of competence itself. It is this sufficiency threshold that proponents of risk-relativity in the determination of competence want to handle flexibly whereas their opponents advocate a fixed, i.e. risk-independent threshold.

### 10.2.3 Competence and Rationality

Impaired decision-making capacities can lead to irrational choices. The latter can, according to the AA-model of legitimate consent, possibly be overridden in order to protect patients from harm due to incompetence. To characterize a decision as 'irrational' can, however, be understood in three distinct ways – inviting for normative misunderstanding and controversy that can only gain from more conceptual differentiation.

In its most narrow understanding decisional irrationality results from a deficit in the capacity to perform *procedurally* correct deliberations (drawing logically correct conclusions etc.). Here, irrationality does indeed correspond to a subset of incompetence. Quite a number of authors take this way, e.g. lawyer-ethicist Larry Alexander:

> If one's choice [...] is to count as valid consent, one must presumably be of a certain *age*, lack serious *mental disease, irrationality*, or *intoxication*, and have a certain degree of *self-control*. (Alexander 1996, p.166ff )

Irrational decisions in this dispositional-procedural sense lack a necessary condition for authority. Thus, if they prove immune against consultation and are prone to appreciably harm the patient they can be disregarded.

A very different concept of irrationality, however, refers *only* to the decision's content. In particular, well-minded physicians have long tended to regard as irrational those patient-decisions that seem incompatible with widely shared values, e.g. decisions to refuse life-saving treatment under certain conditions. According to the depicted standard AA-view, irrationality in this sense of *substantive* deviation from what others consider objectively good or *reasonable* can never serve as a

---

changing nature of the field. Clinical methods and tests to assess capacity are proliferating. The law is also increasingly being called upon to respond to these clinical developments. All of this makes for a very eclectic and challenging field of inquiry." (Charland 2015, sec. 1).

[14] I do not here take issue with questions of the exact nature – gradual or binary, actual or dispositional – of each capability at stake.

justification to override a patient's decision. Otherwise, broadly accepted rights to personalized value-judgements and to their authority would be violated. This danger of undermining patient autonomy by overstretching the concepts of irrationality and competence has long been recognized. It has caused various authors to insist on a strictly *procedural* – in contrast to an *outcome* oriented – understanding at least of competence, if not also of rationality.[15]

Yet another conceptual strategy to block an outcome-based understanding of competence is to describe competence assessment in the practice of informed consent procedures as "gatekeeper". (Beauchamp and Childress 2019, p.112). This already introduced metaphor reflects the view, that competence is in principle *independent* of particular decisions' outcome: Whenever a patient is determined incompetent to make a pending decision, the informed-consent 'game' is over and some surrogate's decision must be sought. To be sure, in many cases, it will still be important and necessary to inform the patient about her condition and treatment alternatives, to assess her preferences, and to deliberate together (see below 10.5.3). But the goal of seeking and relying on *her* treatment authorization must be dispensed with, whenever the patient is 'kept off the gate'.

Between the two depicted options of understanding competence/rationality as dispositional-procedural or else as outcome-oriented in an objective sense, there is, however, a third option that does not fit into the standard binary model of process/outcome views. Probably, it touches the most contested issue in this context, namely the authority of patients' decisions whose content turns out *subjectively* unreasonable, i.e. incompatible with the decision-maker's *own* values. Whether or not you call such decisions irrational,[16] doesn't – as Jason Hanna has recently unfolded and argued for – their "imprudence" resulting from a somewhat "impaired" decision-making undermine their validity as much as is admitted in cases of decisions under obvious pain or emotional distress?[17] Answers to this problem require a deeper analysis of the normative differences between a dispositional and an actual-use understanding of competence/rationality – a task that I must leave to another occasion.

---

[15] So, for instance, Buchanan and Brock (1989, p. 50): "An adequate standard of competence will focus primarily not on the conent of the patient's decision but on the *process* of the reasoning that leads up to that decision." Feinberg (1989, pp.106ff) has insisted on differentiating between a decision's "rationality" in the procedural sense and its "reasonableness", obviously without having been followed.

[16] Thus e.g. Culver and Gert (1990) write: "If one requires a patient to *make use* of his competence when making a decision, the one is no longer judging the competence of the person to decide, but the rationality of the decision made" (p.622; emphasis added).

[17] Compare for instance Hanna 2011. A plausible answer might refer to some surplus value of a policy that insists on the normative difference between impairment and imprudence, even if it cannot be justified in single cases.

### 10.2.4 *Task-Specificity*

Yet another agreed-upon assumption of the standard view on patients' competence is its task-specificity. In the words of Culver and Gert:

> To discuss competence with precision one should focus on a person's competence to do a particular kind of action or make a particular kind of decision, rather than trying to characterize the person as a whole. […] However, even this is too wide a classification, for a person may be competent to make one kind of medical decision and not another kind. (Culver and Gert 1990, p.620)

Assuming *some* task-specificity for patients' decision-making competence is indeed highly plausible for at least two reasons that I will soon discuss. Nevertheless, fine-graining the context-dependence of competence requirements should only go as far as can reasonably be justified. In particular, the task-specificity 'doctrine' and its prima facie plausibility should not be taken as carte blanche for RRCC by simply claiming a medical decision's degree of riskiness to be one of its relevant task-specific aspects.

These are the two arguments in favour of task-specificity: The first is a *general* feature of the very concept of competence. Depending on the task in question, criteria of competence gain strictly different content. Competences to (i) artistically walk on a tightrope[18] or (ii) to consent to one's medical treatment exemplify huge involved differences. Obviously, the first task requires athletic skills, a good sense of balance, and freedom of giddiness whereas the second task requires understanding and evaluating alternative medical risks and benefits for one's own future life within the framework of one's value set.

A second impulse for requiring task-specificity when it comes to patients' medical decision-making results from certain paradigm clinical experiences. Thus, as often discussed, a patient suffering from severe psychotic delusions might prove competent to play chess on a highly competitive level or to make sophisticated financial transactions. But the same patient might be incompetent to evaluate antipsychotic medication, just because she does not realize the pathological nature and provenance of her delusional episodes. Experiences of this type have given rise to medico-legal maxims and regulations not to judge a psychiatric patient *per se* as lacking decisional competency, but to determine her competence with an eye on the specific decisional task she is facing. (Ganzini et al. 2004)

In addition, caretakers are aware that patients' competence may fluctuate according to their emotional conditions: decreasing when they are in a state of pain, anxiety, or excitement and increasing when they feel relaxed and taken care of. Therefore, physicians are commonly advised to regard competency as a context-sensitive phenomenon and to strive as much as possible for optimal conditions when seeking a patient's informed consent. Unquestionably, awareness regarding the context-dependent fragility of patient competence is important. But it goes without

[18] Tightrope walking as a comparative example for understanding competence has been introduced into the RRCC debate by Wilks (1997, p.419ff.). As others have consequently done, I will stick to it.

argument that context-regarding and task-regarding relativity can in principle be kept and handled apart.[19] Thus, context-dependent fragility of cognitive capabilities is a different issue than their task-specificity, though they might look adjacent on first sight. Moreover, to acknowledge that the capabilities making up for someone's competency are decisively task-specific (high wire competence differing from decisional competence) does not solve the problem of how finely these tasks should be *individuated*. This will turn out to be an important point for the risk-relativity issue of decisional competence.

### 10.2.5 The Idea of a Risk-Related Concept of Competence

Take the following example from a recent clinical paper, meant to inform and educate physicians about the understanding and assessment of patients' decision-making capacities:

> [A] mildly demented patient might be able to decide that she wants antibiotic treatment for a urinary tract infection because the treatment allows her to pursue important goals such as feeling well or staying out of the hospital, and its burdens and risks are low. On the other hand, the same patient might be unable to weigh the multiple risks and benefits of a complex neurosurgical procedure with uncertain trade-offs between quality and quantity of life. (Ganzini et al. 2004, p.264)

Obviously, the example is meant to illustrate the view that a patient's competence (here: her being "able") to decide on medical treatments ought to be assessed relative to the "burdens and risks" involved in the decision at stake. The example suggests that a given cognitively impaired patient might be competent to authorize a low-risk antibiotic treatment while not being competent to authorize neurosurgery. Note, however, that the example remains somewhat ambiguous on two points that will later come up for discussion: First, it does not say whether the patient should also be considered competent to *refuse* the antibiotic treatment (most probably not), whereas her asserted decisional incompetence regarding neurosurgery seems to refer to both consent and refusing. Second, the depicted scenario remains unclear as to whether the patient is deemed incompetent to decide about neurosurgery because of the *complexity* of the involved harms and risks of the procedure or rather because of *its degree of riskiness* (probably the latter).

In any case, accepting a risk-relative conception of competence (RRCC) seems to correspond well with widely shared intuitions and to reflect common clinical practice. Moreover, RRCC has to the best of my impressions become an accepted view in bioethics and a – if not *the* – standard model in clinical care.[20] Before start-

[19] Beauchamp seems to overlook this point when he equates "the specific competence to make a certain kind of decision – e.g., whether to cease a certain drug therapy" with "the capacity to *make* such choices in the circumstances" (Beauchamp 1991, p.61).

[20] This view is shared e.g. by Checkland 2001, p.36. Most notably and influentially since Drane's pioneering article, Dan Brock and Allen Buchanan have at length defended RRCC (Buchanan and

ing to critically analyze various arguments for and against this view, I must pay some attention to the general understanding and function of competence judgments in the particular context of patient care. As it will turn out, this understanding already is by no means uncontroversial, although crucial for the RCCT debate.

In his seminal paper, James Drane (1985) suggested three differently demanding standards of patient competence that should be applied in accordance with the quality and probability of harmful consequences of the decisions to be authorized. Thus, he argued for:

(a) A low standard of competence vis-à-vis decisions involving small risks and high benefit. This low standard, he suggested, would already be met whenever a patient is conscious and in possession of any ability to express consent, if only implicitly.
(b) A middle standard of decisional abilities for choosing treatments with high risks of harm if they are a patient's only chance to get better or to survive. This standard could be met by patients who can understand their medical situation and the proposed treatment but who are unable to critically reflect and evaluate options in light of their values and beliefs. Drane suggests that mildly cognitively impaired or borderline patients be among the candidates here.
(c) A high standard of decisional abilities for refusing interventions of low risk and high benefit. Here Drane (1985, p.19) thinks that candidates must be reflective and self-critical and well as in possession of "mature coping devices".

For matters of illustration and simplicity let us fill the categories of treatment in Drane's three standards with the treatment options involved in the example from Sect. 10.1 above: antibiotic treatment for a urinary tract infection as a small risk/high benefit option and complex neurosurgery as a high risk/unclear benefit decision. Thus Drane would have us, for instance, accept a severely demented patient authorizing the antibiotic treatment, but not refusing it. Basically, Drane adduced two arguments, though not in much detail: the moral duty to properly balance respect for autonomy with patient benefit and common clinical practice. The last point is easy to imagine but hard to evidence, and it is certainly not a convincing argument for anybody who considers such practice faulty. The moral argument will be discussed below.

Brock, *Deciding for Others*, Chap. 1). In contrast, Tom Beauchamp and Jim Childress have in their common monograph *Principles of Biomedical Ethics* supported a fixed threshold from the first edition (1979) to the latest one (2019). Remarkably though, Beauchamp has, in his singly authored essay "Competence" (1992), defended RRCC. For a recent RRCC-approval in research consent see Bromwich and Rid 2015. For a recent example from the German-speaking literature see Hermann et al. 2016.

## 10.3 Arguments from Conceptual Grammar

Some authors, such as Tom Beauchamp (1991, pp. 50ff), have tried to draw conceptual conclusions regarding RRCC from what they see as the *general* concept of competence. The underlying assumption is that there is a core concept with a general structure that is prior and transferrable to its contextualized subtypes. In particular, this is playing a role in arguments on normativity, externalism, symmetry, and risk-relativity. As I will try to argue, the idea of a deeper conceptual logic that might answer the controversy on RRCC is implausible. Rather, questions have to be answered within the context of decision-making competences (Likewise, Checkland 2001, p.51).

### *10.3.1 Externalism and Normativity*

Some authors have disputed whether referring to competence's generally *externalist* rather than *internalist* concept can defend RRCC. In the words of Ian Wilks:

> Competence is not an absolute, not a feature solely native and *internal* to a person; competence to render a decision likewise is determined only partly by the qualities of mind that figure in the act. The nature of the options, with their benefits and risks, is also relevant; and this is very much the insight now supplied by those who justify a risk-related standard. (Wilks 1997, p.426)

Although some opponents of RRCC agree with this diagnosis (e.g. Culver and Gert 1990, p.635), the point seems to be poorly made: could anybody seriously deny that capabilities can be purely *internally* realized and at the same time be individualized by an *external* task? (Likewise, Wicclair 1999, p.151) Actually, this seems to be the standard case – as can be exemplified by the capability to distinguish between various shades of grey, to perform tightrope dance over a distance of 100 meters, or to make a decision about medical treatment. Hence, the distinction between internalism and externalism in this sense seems of little help. What is ultimately needed to justify or reject RRCC will be a specification of the external task in question.

In the literature on decisional competence in medical contexts, it is often and rightly emphasized that this concept – like many other competences: even the one in high wire artistry – is *normatively* impregnated. This is by no means a general conceptual feature. Rather, certain circumscribed competences, e.g. the one to correctly memorize 100 digits in a row, are purely descriptive. Normativity comes into play whenever the task in question gets more abstract, allowing for gradual competence or for leeway in choosing and weighing relevant sub-competencies. In such constellations, competence is used as an evaluative résumé of someone's abilities or skills to perform a certain task. It involves three steps, namely (1) the *identification* of the relevant capabilities, (2) a determination of the *degree* to which these abilities are required, and (3) a personalized assessment of someone's possession of these requirements. The first two steps are prone to controversies resulting from dissenting views on the task in question. Thus, there seems to be some latitude, e.g. in deciding whether a (sufficiently) competent high wire artist needs jumping competence or whether the fact that he might be unable to perform for longer than 10 min is of relevance. Whereas athletic competences involve aesthetic values, decisional competence in the context of informed consent involves ethical norms considered relevant for making authoritative decisions. Only the ascriptive third step, certifying the absence or presence of what has been fixed by the first two steps, is by itself non-normative: a given patient is described as meeting or not meeting agreed-upon standards. But, again, *their* nature and degree are set with an eye to their normative function. In Tom Beauchamp's words:

> […] Any concept that serves this function is inherently normative in the way it is used to *establish the abilities and level of abilities* – a normative choice of entry criteria – and to certify a person who possesses such abilities. […] Thus, it is a mistake to infer that empirical judgments of psychological competence are free of prior evaluative commitments. The reverse is true: they are inescapably value laden. (Beauchamp 1991, p.53)

Setting due thresholds for patients' decision-making competence is ruled by two ethical norms: preventing patients from taking decisional responsibility without being 'fit' to do so on one side and preventing the infringement of the rights of 'fit' patients to authorize treatment as they like, on the other side.

Having said this, one crucial problem seems to evolve: Is there a clear distinction to be drawn between competence assessment *motivated* from those two norms as described by the last sentences, and competence assessment *incorporating* a balance of those two norms as RRCC proponents have it? I will come back to this point in Sects. 10.4 and 10.5. But here is already a short anticipatory answer: The *incorporating* (RRCC-) approach seeks to give more weight to beneficence than liberals want to, and it does so in a non-transparent, uninformative way. In contrast, the *motivated* (fixed threshold) approach is bent to explain what grounds legitimate claims to authority. Although a motivated approach can also be applied in a way that violates authority claims, these can only be overridden by blatantly giving priority to beneficence-concerns.

Understanding patient competence as a normative concept is part of the more complex story of what it means to understand authorizing autonomy (AA), the overarching concept, as normative, too. If someone qualifies as an agent of sufficient (task-specific) AA, third parties have good *pro tanto* reasons not to interfere with his self-regarding decision-making. Thus, autonomy and its 'ingredients' are normative in this first sense of constraining third party behaviour. At the same time, they are conceptually and empirically constrained by *why*, depending on rival moral theories, AA is viewed as a claim right to be respected or as a value to be promoted in people's life, at least in our culture. The most straightforward and simplest answer points to AA's instrumental value in shaping one's life according to personal values and preferences as well as to a widespread preference for being in control as such. Both aspects would preclude, e.g., respect for 'authorizations' resulting from drunkenness, error, or manipulation. In this second sense, competence and AA are normative in that they inherit constraints by the very idea of what turns AA into an ingredient of a good life.

### *10.3.2 Asymmetrical Risk-Related Competences?*

Drane's suggestion openly invites a remarkable asymmetry in the authoritative power granted to a given patient: lacking the proposed high standard (see above), she might be considered competent to consent to a certain intervention but incompetent to refuse it, or vice-versa. This asymmetrical competence has been repeatedly rebutted as paradoxical by some (Cale 1999; Demarco 2002, p.234; Hartogh 2016; Wicclair 1991, 1999), but also explicitly been defended by others (Buchanan and Brock 1990; Wilks 1999). As I will try to argue in this and the following section, only the former view is convincing.

It was ethicist Ian Wilks (1997, 1999) who introduced the example of two tightrope walkers into the debate on RRCC in order to defend the latter despite its implication of asymmetrical competence. He makes us imagine two persons facing the challenges of tightrope walking. In Wilks' scenario, one of them does a marvelous artistic job and can thus be called competent to walk on a high line with or without safety net. In contrast, the second candidate happens to still be a rather lousy high wire performer, thus facing a substantial risk that he might fall off the line. According to Wilks, one correctly uses the concept of competence if one describes this second guy as incompetent to perform the high-wire act *without* safety net, but as competent to perform with the net in place. As Wilks asks and then concludes,

> What is the *basis* for the fallible walker's being competent to walk the wire with the net in place, but not without? It is certainly not something intrinsic to the person, not a matter of the person's abilities – since by the terms of the example, there is an equal chance that the fallible walker will complete the task successfully whether the net is in present or not [...]. The difference lies entirely in something extrinsic to the person, in the level of risk the situation involves; and what emerges here is that the level of competence is affected not only by degree of ability but *also* by degree of risk. (Wilks 1997, p.420)

Drawing from various authors' critical answers to Wilks proposal[21], it seems obvious that in his case four different tasks-specific competences can be helpfully distinguished, i.e. the competence to (i) tightrope walking in general; (ii) walk a particular high line without a substantial risk of falling off; (iii) manage the same high line with a safety net in place (unknown to him), possibly interrupted by a drop-off; (iv) take responsibility for walking the high line without a safety net. Wilks' imagined lousy artist lacks (i) and (ii), but possesses (iii); and we are left ignorant about (iv). What then does this case prove?

Competence (i) is a resumé evaluation depending on an artistic candidate's courage together with sophisticated acrobatic skills such as strength, body control, and

[21] Thus, I draw insights from Cale 1999; DeMarco 2002; Checkland 2001, and Wicclair 1999.

balance management. Normally, possession of (i) is *indicated* by a comparatively low risk of falling off the line and thus of risking injury when performing *without* safety net, i.e. competence (ii). (Wicclair 1999) In contrast, if someone has only mediocre acrobatic skills, he will surely lack (i) and (ii) in a package, but might nevertheless possess competence (iii), as in Wilks' example: he might possibly drop off the line but still get credit for mediocre performance. Contrary to Wilk's own description, what makes the mediocre guy competent enough for (iii), but incompetent for (ii) is his relative deficit in genuine ('internal') *abilities* when compared to the other, more brilliant high wire candidate. Competence (ii) for the risky task presupposes high artistic skills (i), while competence (iii) for the comparatively low-risk task does not. Hence, the lesson seems to be that competence-ascriptions might indeed depend on the whether the task in question involves running or avoiding certain risks; in such cases differences in competence can then be reduced to differences in relevant abilities. As with regard to other competences, their ascription depends on the exact nature of the task in question. This might simply become invisible if one attests the mediocre guy's substantial tightrope competence when it comes to performing *with* a net and insufficient tightrope competence when the net is removed.

Moreover, Wilks' analogy would, as others have already argued, be a more appropriate test case for RRCC in medical decision-making if it turned on an acrobatic candidate's *decision* to perform without the safety in question. (Checkland 2001, p.49ff.; Wicclair 1991, p.97ff, and 1999, p.151ff.) Obviously, this decisional competence would depend not primarily on acrobatic skills but mainly on the self-critical appraisal of one's acrobatic potential, as well as on understanding and evaluating the harmful consequences of falling including permanent injury or death. In the context of decision-making the central question is whether Wilks is justified in claiming that:

> [...] cases do indeed exist where one can be competent to say yes but not no, or vice versa; and that it is thus not an anomaly in the risk-related standard [i.e. RRCC] that it entails the existence of such cases. (Wilks 1997, p.413)

Let us then take closer looks at this particular context.

### *10.3.3 Asymmetrical Decisional Competences?*

On first sight, making an informed choice for or against a medical treatment T seems to be an essentially comparative task within a set of options.[22] In the simplest case, the choice is only between T and non-T. In this scenario, understanding and evaluation of risks and benefits *must* count on both sides, because chances of benefit

[22] Epistemically this seems true even in light of a common asymmetry in consent versus refusal *practice*, where the former is taken to require substantial understanding of the relevant facts and prognoses whereas the latter goes without much ado.

from T correspond to risks of non-benefit/harm from non-T. But also in more complex cases e.g. with options T1, T2, or no treatment, evaluation in any reasonable sense involves comparison, i.e. appraisal of each option in the light of its available alternatives.

However, as plausible as a symmetry requirement seems to be in the specific case of patients' informed decision-making for or against treatment options, this might not be true for decision-making competences in other contexts. What can be made of such arguments resulting from examples of the following kind? Take a European politician who is asked to take over major responsibility in nuclear energy politics right after the Fukushima catastrophe. Given her second-order knowledge that she lacks the relevant knowledge and expertise (and maybe even the competence to ever grasp the complex relevant facts) she decides against the offer.[23] Uncontested, she is competent to do so; but had she also been competent to decide the other way? Given the politician's lack of expertise on nuclear dangers, presupposed in the example, one might be tempted to deny this.

On closer sight, this conclusion in favour of an asymmetrical decision competence seems flawed, nonetheless. First of all, the decision on taking over responsibility for nuclear politics is clearly a different one than any decision on how to make use of this responsibility. Second, whatever the outcome of the decision *on* assuming responsibility, it must be based on the *competence* to roughly understand and appraise its necessary preconditions and its possible consequences in both, magnitude and quality. She must, in other words be competent to compare an affirmative and a negative answer and decide in light of this comparison. Therefore, someone who is competent to answer in the affirmative must also be competent to answer no – although her ignorance might be asymmetrical.

Following these arguments, RRCC so far turns implausible only in one of two possible readings. Thus, it does seem implausible that a patient might – as Drane or Brock/Buchanan see it – at the same time be competent to consent to treatment T, but incompetent to refuse T. Here the alleged asymmetry is *choice*-dependent. However, according to a second possible reading of RRCC the granted asymmetry is *choice-set*-dependent.[24] Under this version, a patient might be competent to authorize or refuse treatments whenever *all* options involve only low risk and low hazard, e.g. taking or not taking nose drops to alleviate symptoms of a simple cold. At the same time she might be incompetent to decide for or against *any* available treatment options for a severe neurological damage. Let us look at this *choice-set*-dependent reading of RRCC in the next section.

---

[23] Compare Checkland 2001, p.41ff. on the complex role of second-order abilities in matters of competence.

[24] To my knowledge, in the RRCC literature this distinction has not been systematically pursued.

## 10.4 Arguments from the Task at Stake

Taking stock of the analysis so far, patients' medical decision-making competence is to be determined by the task in question. Thus, understanding and individuating the latter is of decisive importance. Hence, what exactly is the leading idea of granting patients authority over their medical treatment?

### *10.4.1 Making Treatment Preferences Decisive*

Granting authority rights to patients is a special case of granting *rights* to persons. Rights in turn get justified in various ways – much dependent on various legal/ethical theories. Circumventing much of the involved controversies, there seems to be common ground for assuming that patients' authority-rights function (whether primarily or not) as instruments that protect their *interests* in choosing treatment options within the available choice set. The availability in question being determined by factual accessibility and professional standards, patients have to agree or refuse according to their values and preferences.

The importance attributed to *personal* decision-making can be analysed as a threefold one: (i) some medical aspects of an intervention (especially, but not only: pain) can be experienced in personally different ways and degrees, therefore demanding an individual assessment; (ii) generally wanted as well as generally unwanted medical aspects of a given treatment (especially, but not only: end-of-life issues) can have inter-individually different impact on patients' general preferences and thus need individual assessment. I will call this the *life-shaping*[25] or *holistic* aspects that some medical decisions might have; (iii) being treated as an authorizer over one's medical treatment has in our culture become *as such* an aspect of being respectfully treated as a person.

Trivially true but easily forgotten, the tasks in question are very different from physicians' tasks to come up with treatment recommendations in the first place: with regard to medical chances and risks, the patient's part is usually and inevitably that of a lay-user who has to rely on expert opinion, thus making various and again often implicit judgments on the expert's trustworthiness, on the information she considers pertinent, and on the treatment's potential impact on her life. Where this might be a simple task at the dentist who recommends refilling a back tooth, it might become complex in other contexts. Here, medical decision-making can, as already emphasized, gain the importance of *life-shaping* – in light of a patient's personal fears, hopes, values, or preferences that might well turn her into a 'non-standard' patient.

Hence, decisions about medical options might gain what I have called a holistic dimension. This is particularly likely, if such decisions might have substantial

[25] This – somewhat self-imposing – expression is owed to Silver (2002, p.462ff.).

effects on one's quality or length of life – as in matters of reproduction, body shape or mental states, research settings for the treatment of major ailments, or end-of-life scenarios. Even here, life shaping is, of course, partial, given the many natural and social determinants of a human life. Moreover, life shaping neither needs to be ambitious, nor explicit, nor even positively wanted. But it is always an option to some extent, even if produced by negative decisions. Last not least, life shaping in the explained sense is an option not supported by all *cultures* (cf. Beauchamp 1991, p.59ff.).

Given this trivial reminder, it should become clear that self-regarding medical decision-making might get *a* holistic, and value-laden dimension going far beyond the professional expertise of physicians. To perform this task, patients need to understand such core concepts as life, disease, death, and risk. They must have 'ordinary' computational skills, a decent memory, and the ability to deliberate. And they must have some evaluative framework relative to which they can appreciate and comparatively evaluate treatment different burdens, benefits, and life perspectives.

Obviously, these deliberations add nothing *really* new to the standard view of patient competence as a set of mental abilities (see Sect. 10.2). It might only make clearer that patient competency has to *differ* from other decisional competences – e.g. from physicians' competence for identifying best treatment options or from people's competence for risk assessment in various other private or professional realms contexts – mainly by its *personal evaluative holism*. This might also explain some of the ongoing controversies in bioethics about the proper conceptual place of personal values and personal value-conformity ('authenticity') in informed consent, because this place is often not sufficiently elaborated in the standard view.[26]

### *10.4.2 The Ordinary-Person Standard*

Holistic decision-makers about medical treatments, I have suggested, do need a set of values and sufficient understanding of such key concepts as disease and death, risk and probability, uncertainties, of expertise and credibility. They need the ability to understand something about risk framing and to appreciate the potential occurrence of specific harms and benefits for their lives. But none of these requirements exceeds the competences of an ordinary person. This thesis does not follow from any empirical data showing that ordinary persons happen to have the competencies

[26] See Sect. 10.2.2. above. Sometimes reference to values is made within the bundle of mental capacities, e.g. requiring "the ability [...] to evaluate [treatment] consequences in view of one's own values" (Hartogh 2016, p.71) – presupposing the possession of such values. Sometimes authenticity is introduced as an additional requirement outside (narrowly understood) competency, see (Quante 2011). Value conformity should not get misunderstood as nailing patients down to their past values: As has often been emphasized, it should also entail leeway for new, may be 'courageous' evaluations.

in question. Rather, it follows from the normative premise that competence requirements standards *should* be governed by an ordinary person standard. After all, it is normal people who are viewed as giving shape and meaning to their lives, not some extraordinarily gifted sub-class of them.[27]

So far, nothing in this section has explicitly touched the main issue of RRCC, namely whether risky choice-sets (e.g., decisions for or against neurosurgery) do not, after all, require some deeper competence in grasping these decisions' potential life-shaping meaning than do low-risk choice sets (e.g., regular decisions at the dentist). But now, this suggestion can clearly be dismissed: What is needed in either scenario is a somewhat realistic assessment of the decisions' degree of riskiness and of riskiness as such: In order to meet AA requirements, a patient at the dentist must be competent to understand the relative *absence* of risk (and the latter's meaning). Likewise, the patient to whom neurosurgery has been recommended must be competent to understand the relative *presence* of risk and what this means for life and health and maybe for his life-plans etc. Hence, to assess some treatments as trivial and others as non-trivial for one's life-shaping project presupposes the very same basic competences.

On the other hand, there are many decision-makers who do not qualify for evaluative holism and thus do not count as competent decision-makers, even if the issues at stake are completely trivial. Of course, a severely demented patient might and should be respected in as many of their self-regarding choices on trivial matters or harmless issues as possible. But this should not blur important distinctions in justifying *why* someone's decisions should be respected (see Sect. 5.4 below).

### *10.4.3 Complex* **Versus** *Risky Decisions*

A controversially answered question in the RRCC debate concerns the role of certain medical issues' *complexity*. This complexity, it is sometimes argued, might in certain cases require beyond-ordinary cognitive skills, but should be kept apart from riskiness. In Beauchamp/Childress' words:

> It is correct to say that the level of a person's capacity to decide will rise as the *complexity* or *difficulty* of a task increases (deciding about spinal fusion, say, as contrasted with deciding whether to take a minor tranquilizer), but the level of competence to decide does not rise as the *risk* of an outcome increases. It is confusing to blend a decision's complexity or difficulty with the risk at stake. (Beauchamp and Childress 2019, p.117)

Convincing as this seems on first sight and in principle, I tend to think that a *complexity*-relative concept of competence will rarely, if ever, be relevant and that the opposite view might rest on a misunderstanding: to make holistic evaluations, patients do *not* have to understand why and by which mechanisms a spinal fusion or

[27] This view, I take it, belongs to the framing theses of the AA-model of informed consent. Compare Beauchamp and Childress 2019, p.100ff.

rather a tranquilizer might or might not be effective. Rather, they have to understand a procedure's chances of cure, its uncertainties or possibly its being a non-stand procedure. Ordinary persons, I take it, can grasp such aspects if they are communicated understandably. Physicians' communication about complex treatment and about its expected consequences plays a major role in empowering patients to become autonomous authorizers. The task of translating science talk into messages that ordinary patients can understand remains a challenge. The same proves true for risk communication, which has been shown to lead to innumerable false beliefs on the part of patients. But ultimately this seems a matter of deficit understanding and incompetent communication on the side of physicians rather than a lack of capabilities on the part of patients (See Gigerenzer et al. 2007).

## 10.5 Arguments from Protection

### *10.5.1 Fallibilism: Raising Standards of Evidence or of Substance?*

Paying particular attention to a patient's competence whenever she wants to choose *against* recommended treatments has already been identified (see Sect. 10.2.1) as a prudent strategy in the service of detecting incompetence at low moral cost. The same is true for paying closer attention to a patient's competence whenever the choice-set involves considerable risks of harm in absolute terms – *regardless* of physicians' recommendations. In both cases not competence itself but *evidence* of competence is subject to stricter requirements in case of risk-taking decisions. Many have thus recommended this 'ethically innocent' precautionary policy (e.g. Beauchamp and Childress 2019, p.117f.; Wicclair 1999, p.153).

Obviously, raising the standards of *evidence* of competence for risky choices principally differs from raising the *substantive* standards of competence, i.e. in *degree or quality*. However, Joel Feinberg, pioneering proponent of respecting personal autonomy in both law and ethics, has tried to *link* the two in defending RRCC on what he sees as purely fallibilistic or epistemic ground:

> *The more risky the conduct the greater the degree of voluntariness required if the conduct is to be permitted.* [...] [This] entails that the voluntariness required for permissible self-endangering actions should be determined by standards whose stringency varies directly with the gravity of the risked harm and with the probability of the risked harm occurring. (Feinberg 1989, pp.118/1190)

Bioethicists Brock and Buchanan (1989, p.45ff.) who accuse Feinberg of hidden, though unwanted paternalism, have famously criticized his argument. In a nutshell they argue that any RRCC-policy will have two simultaneous effects: it will (i) protect some patients from the harm of risky, though incompetent decisions (the wanted effect), but it will also (ii) violate the autonomy of some other patients who falsely get assessed as incompetent (the unwanted, but accepted side effect). Accepting (ii) as the moral price for (i), so Brock and Buchanan's argument, can only be justified from a position that ultimately ranks the reduction of harm by effect (i) morally higher than the violation of autonomy by effect (ii) – a (paternalist) position that they themselves favor anyhow and explicitly.

On closer analysis,[28] Feinberg's suggestion cannot be as easily dismissed as Brock/Buchanan have it, but it seems unconvincing, nevertheless. A Feinberg-style strategy can indeed – and against Brock/Buchanan – be reconstructed as compatible with giving first priority to the protection of autonomy over harm. Hence, with an eye on policy-making the strategy might be justified in contexts with genuine *uncertainty* about the nature of the required competence and with a sufficiently high probability that severe harm from incompetent decision-making can indeed be prevented by effect (ii). From an *ex ante* view of uncertainty, a high likelihood of non-autonomously chosen harm can then outweigh a smaller likelihood of violating autonomy although respect for autonomy gets clear lexical priority over the prevention of autonomously self-afflicted harm.[29] *Ex post*, an analogous balance would hold true for collectives of persons so treated: many cases of prevented non-autonomously chosen harm might outweigh rare cases of violated autonomy. Given that the latter cannot be identified in advance, even proponents of inviolable autonomy rights might swallow this.[30] In such contexts, a policy of raising standards (and tests) might be justified on clearly autonomy-oriented grounds. These grounds, that is, do *not* require neglecting the prevention of harm, especially if unauthorized, in the moral calculus, only to rank it second place.[31]

But again, granting this presupposes circumstances of genuine conceptual uncertainty and appropriate proportionality. Both conditions seem to be *missing* in the context of medical decision-making. Here we *know* that ordinary persons' competence is sufficient and that requiring *more* than this will thus *always* result in violation of autonomous authorization and often in the prevention of 'harm' that, given the choice-set available to them, patients themselves assess as minor evils. Therefore, RRCC does *not* seem justifiable on fallibilistic grounds.

---

[28] I find myself in some agreement with and owe much to ethicist Joseph Demarco (2002) who first drew my attention to this particular debate.

[29] Compare Demarco 2002, p.236ff.

[30] Systematically, Feinberg's position falls under what Fateh-Moghadan and Gutmann have labeled the "endangerment"-variety of soft paternalism. They, too, rightly stress the importance of "proportionality" in justifying such policies and their inherent danger of hidden hard paternalism (Fateh-Moghadam and Gutmann 2014, p.392ff.).

[31] This is what Buchanan/Brock seem, however, to require from a non-paternalist position: compare Buchanan and Brock 1989, p.41ff.

### 10.5.2 Over-Exclusiveness: Hidden Paternalism

From a critical perspective, favoring RRCC can have both over-*exclusive* and over-*inclusive* motivations and consequences. Thus, it aims at (i) protecting patients, even if they might be competent according to the ordinary-person standard, against self-regarding decisions that from outside are deemed gravely harmful. And it is ready to (ii) grant decision-making authority to patients far *below* that standard as long as their decisions involve low-risk issues. Whether someone's pro-RRCC intuitions are more in line with (i) or with (ii), the two sides of the coin might well coincide as *two* mutually supportive lines of argument. I will briefly discuss the first one in this section and the second one thereafter.

Anti-paternalism holds that a competent patient's voluntary and informed decision should never be overridden so as to protect him from harm. In this paper there is no room to discuss paternalism and anti-paternalism in their own right. However, as several critics have warned, introducing RRCC turns

> [...] the statement that a competent patient's decision may not be overridden for paternalistic reasons [into] a tautology rather than an expression of an important liberal-democratic principle. (Wicclair 1999, p. 150)

This conclusion is correct because RRCC is *masking* whether a patient's decision has been overridden due to 'real' incompetence or rather with an eye on impeding self-afflicted harm. This is especially true since RRCC-proponents do not (and probably cannot) give full particulars about what exactly they require for sufficient competence in cases of (seemingly) hazardous decisions. Rather, it seems conceivable that patients are *never* viewed sufficiently competent to make certain decisions (e.g. suicide).

Paternalists, of course, would not much mind and have explicitly suggested giving up the traditional distinction between the criteria of competence and harm (e.g., Hartogh 2016). But I can only confirm DeMarco's (2002, p. 244) testimony: "Autonomy is too important, and paternalism is too controversial to be buried in a concept of competence."

### 10.5.3 Over-Inclusiveness: Devaluating Authorization

Coming to the other end of the competence scale, including incompetent patients into the sphere of personal *respect* seems to be a major motivation behind RRCC. Many of the underlying concerns can be easily understood: judging a patient incompetent can hurt or stigmatize her. As emphasized for instance by Vandeveer (2014, p.415), it might even function as a 'self-fulfilling prophecy'. Moreover, caretakers might easily forget that the incompetent should be respected as choosers whenever possible, thus enhancing their preference satisfaction and their self-esteem. It is a sad and completely unnecessary story that the attribution of incompetence should lead caregivers to forget their duties of benefiting patients by following their self-regarding choices whenever possible without afflicting major harm.

This might be all the truer, as *over-inclusion* via RRCC would be limited to those decisions that are deemed low-risk/high-benefit in the first place. Hence, only *as-if-authority* or *illusory* autonomy is granted to those patients. For any harmful decision physicians would jump in and take over.

But even then, three serious objections have to be made against the attribution of illusory (or *pseudo-*) autonomy. First, it confounds reasonable concepts of competence, authority, and autonomy, possibly inviting caretakers to lose respect for 'real' autonomy. Secondly, by circumventing the need for transparent surrogate decision-making procedures, RRCC re-opens a back door to paternalism in medicine. And thirdly, respectful over-inclusion might fuel the belief - wrong in my eyes - that severely demented patients can validly revoke their former advance directives. This is a contested issue that cannot be explicated here. Suffice it to hint at the logical connection between RRCC and the 'past-directive-versus-present-interest conflict' in severely demented patients.[32]

Thus, granting pseudo-competence to an incompetent patient might *look* respectful. Explicitly following her wishes in matters that involve only low risk and low harm as well as following her whenever she agrees to a recommended low-risk option surely is the right thing to do. However, doing this under the label of AA intentionally obscures the locus of responsibility and ultimate decision-making (likewise, Wicclair 1991, p.101).

## 10.6 Conclusions

In this paper, I have argued in favor of a *fixed* concept of decisional competence for patients in the context of giving their informed consent to medical treatments. Although its alternative, a risk-relative conception of competence (RRCC), might well have become the governing conception among clinicians and clinical ethicists it runs into fundamental problems. As ethicist DeMarco (2002, p.232) put it about fifteen years ago: "[…] including risk in the definition of 'competence', or even raising the standard of competence due to risk, is a fundamental mistake that obscures proper decision making in bioethics."

I have tried to reaffirm this view by reviewing well-known RRCC-objections from symmetry problems and the dangers of *hidden* paternalism towards patients with uncompromised competence. Moreover, I have argued that RRCC misconceives the specific task behind patient competence, i.e. optionally making medical decisions with an eye on one's shape of life within the boundaries of being *ordinary* women and men. Finally, by attributing illusory autonomy to clearly incompetent

[32] Compare Dworkin 1986; Dresser 1995; Jox et al. 2012; Schoene-Seifert et al. 2016.

patients, RRCC not only obscures the need for surrogate decision making, but it also implies conceptual de-differentiations that turn out highly problematic in other areas of bioethical dispute, e.g. about honoring advance directives against severely demented patients' expressed behavior.

## References


Alexander, Larry. 1996. The Moral Magic of Consent (II). *Legal Theory* 2 (3): 165–174.

Amelung, Knut. 1992. Über die Einwilligungsfähigkeit (Teil I). *Zeitschrift für die gesamte Strafrechtswissenschaft* 3: 525–558.

Beauchamp, Tom L. 1991. Competence. In *Competency. A Study of Informal Competency Determinations in Primary Care*, ed. Mary Ann Gardell Cutter and Earl E. Shelp, 49–77. Dordrecht: Springer.

Beauchamp, Tom L., and James F. Childress. 2019. *Principles of Biomedical Ethics*. Vol. 8. New York/Oxford: Oxford University Press.

Bromwich, Danielle, and Annette Rid. 2015. Can Informed Consent to Research Be Adapted to Risk? *Journal of Medical Ethics* 41 (7): 521–528.

Buchanan, Allen E., and Dan W. Brock. 1989. *Deciding for Others: The Ethics of Surrogate Decision Making*. Cambridge: Cambridge University Press.

Cale, Gita S. 1999. Continuing the Debate over Risk-Related Standards of Competence. *Bioethics* 13 (2): 131–148.

Charland, Louis C. 2015. Decision-Making Capacity. In *The Stanford Encyclopedia of Philosophy*, ed. Edward N. Zalta, https://plato.stanford.edu/archives/fall2015/entries/decision-capacity/.

Checkland, David. 2001. On Risk and Decisional Capacity. *Journal of Medicine and Philosophy* 26 (1): 35–59.

Culver, Charles M., and Bernard Gert. 1990. The Inadequacy of Incompetence. *The Milbank Quarterly*: 619–643.

DeMarco, Joseph P. 2002. Competence and Paternalism. *Bioethics* 16 (3): 231–245.

Drane, James F. 1985. The Many Faces of Competency. *Hastings Center Report* 15 (2): 17–21.

Dresser, Rebecca S. 1995. Dworkin on Dementia. Elegant Theory, Questionable Policy. *Hastings Center Report* 25 (6): 32–38.

Dworkin, Ronald. 1986. Autonomy and the Demented Self. *The Milbank Quarterly* 64 (Suppl. 2): 4–16.

Faden, Ruth R., and Tom L. Beauchamp. 1986. *A History and Theory of Informed Consent*. New York/Oxford: Oxford University Press.

Fateh-Moghadam, Bijan, and Thomas Gutmann. 2014. Governing [through] Autonomy. The Moral and Legal Limits of 'Soft Paternalism'. *Ethical Theory and Moral Practice* 17 (3): 383–397.

Feinberg, Joel. 1989. *Moral Limits of the Criminal Law: Harm to Self*. New York/Oxford: Oxford University Press.

Ganzini, Linda, Ladislav Volicer, William A. Nelson, Ellen Fox, and Arthur R. Derse. 2004. Ten Myths about Decision-Making Capacity. *Journal of the American Medical Directors Association* 5 (4): 263–267.

Gaylin, Willard. 1982, April 1. The Competence of Children: No Longer All or None. *Hastings Center Report* 12 (2): 33–38. https://doi.org/10.2307/3561805.

Gigerenzer, Gerd, Wolfgang Gaissmaier, Elke Kurz-Milcke, Lisa M. Schwartz, and Steven Woloshin. 2007. Helping Doctors and Patients Make Sense of Health Statistics. *Psychological Science in the Public Interest* 8 (2): 53–96.

Hanna, Jason. 2011. Paternalism and Impairment. *Social Theory and Practice* 37 (3): 434–460.

Hartogh, Govert den. 2016. Do We Need a Threshold Conception of Competence? *Medicine, Health Care and Philosophy* 19: 71–83. https://doi.org/10.1007/s11019-015-9646-5.

Hermann, Helena, Manuel Trachsel, and Nikola Biller-Andorno. 2016. Decision-Making Capacity: Inherent Ability or Ethical Judgment? *Ethik in der Medizin* 28 (2): 107–120

Jox, Ralf J., et al. 2012. Surrogate Decision Making for Patients with End-Stage Dementia. *International Journal of Geriatric Psychiatry* 27 (10): 1045–1052.

Macklin, Ruth. 1987. *Mortal Choices: Ethical Dilemmas in Modern Medicine*. Boston: Houghton Mifflin.

Manson, Neil C., and Onora O'Neill. 2007. *Rethinking Informed Consent in Bioethics*. Cambridge: Cambridge University Press.

Miller, Franklin G., and Alan Wertheimer. 2011. The Fair Transaction Model of Informed Consent: An Alternative to Autonomous Authorization. *Kennedy Institute of Ethics Journal* 21 (3): 201–218.

Quante, Michael. 2011. In Defence of Personal Autonomy. *Journal of Medical Ethics* 37 (10): 597–600.

Roth, Loren H., Alan Meisel, and Charles W. Lidz. 1977. Tests of Competency to Consent to Treatment. *The American Journal of Psychiatry* 134 (3): 279–284.

Schoene-Seifert, Bettina, Anna Lena Uerpmann, J. Jochaim Gerss, and David Herr. 2016. Advance (Meta-) Directives for Patients with Dementia who Appear Content: Learning from a Nationwide Survey. *Journal of the American Medical Directors Association* 17 (4): 294–299.

Vandeveer, Donald. 2014. *Paternalistic Intervention: The Moral Bounds on Benevolence*. Princeton: Princeton University Press. https://doi.org/10.1515/9781400854066.

Silver, Mitchell. 2002. Reflections On Determining Competency. *Bioethics* 16 (5): 455–468.

Wicclair, Mark R. 1991. Patient Decision-Making Capacity and Risk. *Bioethics* 5 (2): 91–104.

———. 1999. The Continuing Debate over Risk-Related Standards of Competence. *Bioethics* 13 (2): 149–153.

Wilks, Ian. 1997. The Debate over Risk-Related Standards of Competence. *Bioethics* 11 (5): 413–426.

———. 1999. Asymmetrical Competence. *Bioethics* 13 (2): 154–159.

# Chapter 11
# Vulnerability, Exploitation and Autonomy

**Catriona Mackenzie**

**Abstract** Bioethicists who seek to defend commercial transactions that intuitively seem exploitative, such as organ sales and commercial surrogacy, typically pair a liberal analysis of exploitation with a libertarian analysis of autonomy. In this paper, I argue that the liberal analysis of exploitation, which focuses primarily on two party transactions between individuals, occludes the structural dimensions of exploitation. This occlusion then paves the way for the transaction to be understood in terms of libertarian autonomy. I propose that a vulnerability analysis paired with a multidimensional and relational theory of autonomy highlights the structural dimensions of exploitation and exposes the myth-making that underlies claims that these forms of exploitation are autonomy-enhancing.

## 11.1 Introduction

Over the last two decades a growing body of ethnographic research has sought to investigate and give voice to the lived experience of people who have been recruited into the global trade in body parts and reproductive services. Ethnographic research with kidney sellers in Pakistan, Bangladesh, Egypt, Iran, Brazil and the Philippines, amongst other countries, and with gestational surrogates in India, has helped to shed light on these people's socio-economic plight and family situations, their motivations, and the recruitment tactics used by brokers.[1] This research has also painted a disturbing picture of the circumstances in which they undergo surgery or perform reproductive labour, and of their lives in the aftermath of their decisions.

[1] For examples of the ethnographic research conducted with organ sellers in a range of different countries, see Scheper-Hughes (2000, 2008), Moazam et al. (2009), Moniruzzaman (2012). Ethnographic research conducted with surrogates in India is reported in Pande (2010).

C. Mackenzie (✉)
Macquarie University, Sydney, Australia
e-mail: catriona.mackenzie@mq.edu.au



J. F. Childress, M. Quante (eds.), *Thick (Concepts of) Autonomy*, Philosophical Studies Series 146, https://doi.org/10.1007/978-3-030-80991-1_11

Invariably, people recruited as kidney sellers or gestational surrogates are desperately poor, illiterate, indebted, suffer poor nutrition, live in inadequate housing, and have extremely limited options for what they can be and do. The options of surrogates, in addition, are constrained by entrenched patriarchal gender norms. To use the terminology of Jonathon Wolff and Avner de Shalit (2007), those recruited could be characterised as experiencing extreme insecurity of functioning across a range of different functionings. Moreover, especially in the case of kidney sellers, the ethnographic research provides evidence that the vast majority of those recruited regret their decision and subsequently end up being worse off financially, as well as experiencing significant physical, psychological and social suffering.[2] This research therefore suggests that the global trade in body parts and reproductive services is grossly exploitative of extremely disadvantaged and vulnerable persons; it is a noxious market.

Over the same period in which the results of this ethnographic research have been published, there has been a chorus of voices in bioethics arguing in favour of regulated global markets in reproductive services and in nonessential or renewable body parts.[3] Defenders of such markets typically pair a liberal, transactional analysis of exploitation with a libertarian analysis of autonomy. Liberal, transactional accounts, which Jeremy Snyder (2012) refers to as micro fairness accounts, analyse exploitation in terms of impaired consent and/or an unfair bargain, contract or offer.[4] On these views, what makes a specific transaction unfair, and therefore potentially exploitative, is when one party A gains more, or the other party B gains less, than they should from the transaction. The standard of fairness is what would be achieved under hypothetical ideal fair market conditions. To show that organ selling or commercial gestational surrogacy is exploitative thus requires showing that the consent of the seller or surrogate is impaired, or that the bargain or contract is unfair in the sense that the seller or surrogate does not receive a fair share of the benefits of the transaction. It is important to note that the fairness or otherwise of the background social and economic conditions in which the transaction occurs is bracketed from consideration.

Libertarian conceptions of autonomy equate personal autonomy with negative liberty and hold that to be autonomous is to be free from unwarranted external interference by other persons or the state with respect to important decisions about one's life. In bioethics, autonomy theorists of a more libertarian bent operate with a minimalist conception of autonomous decision-making as voluntary and informed choice. They hold that autonomy is best promoted by maximising individual freedom of choice and minimising regulatory and other kinds of constraints on choice.[5]

Pairing the liberal, transactional analysis of exploitation with a libertarian conception of autonomy, the defense of organ markets, for example, typically goes as

---

[2] See Koplin (2014) for a summary of the ethnographic research documenting regret in relation to the decision to sell a kidney.

[3] See e.g. Fabre (2006), Radcliffe-Richard (2007), Taylor (2002), Wilkinson (2003).

[4] Wertheimer (1996) is the classic source for the liberal, transactional account. See also Wertheimer (2011).

[5] In Mackenzie (2015), I provide a more detailed discussion and critique of libertarian conceptions of autonomy in bioethics.

follows. Individuals have an autonomy right to use their bodies however they choose, including selling body parts for material gain. If a seller consents to the sale of her body parts in full knowledge of the potential risks involved, and perceives the financial offer as advantageous and as likely to make her better off relative to her current situation, then the seller has a right to enter into the transaction even if it appears exploitative. This is a case of what Wertheimer (1996, 2011) would call 'mutually advantageous exploitation'. Commercial markets in organs therefore provide prospective sellers with autonomy-enhancing options and prohibiting such sales or other high-risk opportunities for improving their material situation is unjustifiably paternalistic.

My aim in this paper is to argue that the conceptions of autonomy and exploitation assumed in this kind of argument occlude the structural inequalities and injustices that must be central to any adequate assessment of whether so-called mutually advantageous exploitation is autonomy-enhancing.[6] My argument proceeds in three steps. In the first step, I propose that the concepts of situational and pathogenic vulnerability (Mackenzie, Rogers, Dodds 2014) and corrosive disadvantage (Wolff and de Shalit 2007) can help to clarify the sense in which people who make desperate choices to sell kidneys or become gestational surrogates are vulnerable to exploitation. In the second step, I draw on Snyder's (2012) taxonomy of exploitation and Vida Panitch's (2013, 2017) work on transnational commercial surrogacy to show why the transactional or micro fairness account of exploitation is insufficient for addressing the moral question of whether markets in organs and reproductive services are exploitative. In the third step, I propose that a multidimensional and relational analysis of autonomy (Mackenzie 2014) illuminates the different ways that autonomy can be compromised by disadvantage, vulnerability and social oppression. This analysis exposes what I regard as the myth-making in the claim that mutually advantageous exploitation can be autonomy-enhancing. I also endorse a suggestion by Malmqvist (2014), that a group soft paternalist approach to markets in organs and reproductive services might be justified to avoid harms to individuals whose autonomy is likely compromised by disadvantage.

A clarification may be useful at this point. My aim in the paper is to show why the conceptions of exploitation and autonomy assumed by defenders of markets in organs and reproductive services are inadequate. I do not offer a defense of either prohibition or regulation with respect to such markets, although my argument might point in the direction of prohibition as an appropriate policy response. However, since organ selling and transnational gestational surrogacy are distinct practices, the merits of prohibition versus regulation need to be debated separately in each case and with reference to the specificities of the relevant jurisdictional contexts.[7] In

---

[6] The importance of attending to structural injustice for understanding exploitation in a range of practical contexts, including gestational surrogacy and sweatshop labour, is a central theme of many of the essays in Deveaux and Panitch (2017).

[7] In bioethics, the literatures on organ selling and the transnational market in reproductive services are quite distinct. While I acknowledge that these different kinds of market raise distinct moral and policy issues, my aim in discussing them together in this paper is to highlight the structural com-

addition, as Serene Khader (2013) argues, any policy recommendations need to be attentive to an intersectional and context-sensitive analysis of the specific kinds of class or gender harms that might be caused either by such markets or by different kinds of regulatory intervention or prohibition.

## 11.2 Vulnerability and Corrosive Disadvantage

To exploit someone is to take advantage of her vulnerability. How then should vulnerability be analysed? To be vulnerable is to be at increased risk of suffering harm or being wronged.[8] This risk might be potential or occurrent. Hence efforts to mitigate or alleviate a specific vulnerability will need to attend to whether the risk of the person being harmed or wronged is potential or occurrent. For example, poverty can make a person vulnerable to homelessness. If she has become unemployed and has no income, is behind on her rent, and is about to be evicted from her home, then she is occurrently vulnerable to homelessness. If she has some form of precarious employment, but her income is insecure and she struggles to pay the rent and keep up with her bills, then while she is not occurrently vulnerable to homelessness, she is potentially vulnerable to homelessness.

In bioethics there has been considerable debate between two approaches to vulnerability: ontological and relational or context-specific.[9] The taxonomy of different sources of vulnerability that I have developed in earlier work with Wendy Rogers and Susan Dodds, aims to reconcile these two approaches. The example of homelessness is useful for helping to clarify this taxonomy, which distinguishes inherent, situational and pathogenic sources of vulnerability.

The notion of inherent vulnerability acknowledges that vulnerability is an ontological condition of our humanity. We are all inherently vulnerable because we are finite, embodied and social creatures with needs. And it is by virtue of this inherent neediness that we are vulnerable to harm (physical, psychological, emotional) and to being wronged by others. Using the example of homelessness, because one of our basic needs is the need for adequate housing or shelter, all human beings are inherently vulnerable to homelessness.

---

monalities in the types of arguments used by defenders of transnational markets in body parts and reproductive services.

[8] Hurst (2008) analyses vulnerability in terms of increased risk of being subject to wrongful harms. Her reasons for restricting the analysis of vulnerability to wrongful harms rather than harms more broadly are twofold. First, because she is unsympathetic to ontological accounts of vulnerability; and second, to make it easier to identify which duties are required to remediate specific vulnerabilities and on whom those duties fall. However, an implication of her view is that persons cannot be characterised as vulnerable unless their increased risk of harm arises from wrongful actions on the part of others. Thus, persons at increased risk of suffering harm as a result of accidents, natural catastrophes, or illness would not count as vulnerable on this view. This seems counter-intuitive to me and inconsistent with the way the concept of vulnerability is employed in everyday usage.

[9] For more detailed discussion of this debate and of the taxonomy discussed below, see Rogers, Mackenzie, Dodds (2012) and Mackenzie, Rogers, Dodds (2014).

However, clearly we are not all equally vulnerable to homelessness. Further, what counts as adequate housing varies according to context. The notion of situational vulnerability draws attention to the context-specific factors that shape the ways in which vulnerability might be manifested and that might render a person or social group especially vulnerable, in this case to homelessness. Such factors are many and varied and may include environmental conditions, social norms and practices, institutional structures (political, economic, legal), as well as the individual's specific situation or needs. A person who is mobility impaired, for example, and who needs wheelchair accessible housing may be more vulnerable to homelessness than a person who can easily climb several flights of stairs.

The notion of pathogenic vulnerability refers to a sub-set of situational vulnerabilities that are caused by morally dysfunctional, oppressive or dominating social relationships, or by remediable structural inequality and injustice. We also use the term to refer to vulnerabilities that are caused by (sometimes well-intentioned) interventions to remediate vulnerability. A young teenager who was being sexually abused at home by a relative and is now homeless, experiences pathogenic vulnerability. This vulnerability may be further compounded by an intervention designed to remediate that vulnerability, such as housing in a shelter for young people if, for example, she develops a drug addiction or is exposed to further abuse and violence while living in the shelter. This example shows that the distinction between inherent, situational and pathogenic vulnerability is not categorical and that these sources of vulnerability can and often do overlap and interact in complex ways.

The work of Wolff and de Shalit (2007) on corrosive disadvantage is helpful for clarifying the complex interactions between different sources of vulnerability. Wolff and de Shalit analyse disadvantage in terms of insecurity of functioning across a range of functionings.[10] People who are disadvantaged experience not only insecurity of functioning, but also lack genuine opportunities for secure functionings. Moreover, this insecurity and lack of genuine opportunity typically affects not just one functioning but a clustering of functionings, with cumulative effects over time. An example of such clustering is the way over time unemployment can lead to homelessness, and then loss of friendship networks, then ill health (Wolff and de Shalit 2007, 120). The concept of "corrosive disadvantage" refers to the way in which poor or insecure functioning in one domain can cause poor or insecure functionings in other domains, as in this example. Wolff and de Shalit further argue that disadvantage typically exposes people to risks that those who are advantaged do not face and that taking these risks can generate corrosive disadvantage when the risks taken in an attempt to secure one functioning then jeopardises other functionings. They refer to this kind of risk taking as "inverse cross category risk" (70).

Earlier I defined vulnerability as being at increased risk of suffering harm or being wronged. In contexts where vulnerability is associated with disadvantage, it could also be understood as being at increased risk of insecurity of functionings,

[10] Wolff and de Shalit distil Nussbaum's list of ten capabilities into six central functionings: life, bodily health, bodily integrity, affiliation, control over one's environment, and sense, imagination and thought (2007, 106).

where the source of that insecurity is likely to be some combination of inherent, situational and pathogenic vulnerability. In the example of the dynamic clustering over time of unemployment, homelessness, loss of social networks and ill health, the initial situational vulnerability of the unemployed person exposes her to pathogenic forms of vulnerability (homelessness and social isolation), which then increases her inherent vulnerability (illness).

What is abundantly evident from the ethnographic research is that those people who are initially recruited to sell kidneys or to labour as gestational surrogates are pathogenically vulnerable, experience significant insecurity of functionings and lack genuine opportunities for functionings. To describe these people as pathogenically vulnerable is not to deny their agency. It is rather to characterise the structurally unjust and institutionally dysfunctional circumstances in which they exercise agency, circumstances which tempt them to take risks that they would not take if they had genuine alternative opportunities for functioning. In the case of kidney sellers, the risky choice of surgery then exposes them to significant inverse cross-category risk over time: ill health, loss of livelihood, social exclusion, psychological suffering, and deepened financial insecurity.[11]

While defenders of markets in organs acknowledge that, even in a regulated market, those recruited to sell their organs will continue to be the desperately poor, they argue that a regulated market would mitigate some of these additional risks. Whether or not this might be the case is an empirical question. The evidence from Iran (where there has been a regulated market in organs since 1988) suggests otherwise.[12] However, in light of the analysis of vulnerability and disadvantage outlined in this section, it seems fanciful to claim that the availability of the option to sell a kidney or labour as a gestational surrogate is autonomy-enhancing. I return to this issue in section 4. In the next section I focus on the question of exploitation.

## 11.3 Exploitation and Injustice

I noted earlier that exploitation involves taking advantage of another's vulnerability. Vulnerability therefore makes a person potentially exploitable. How should exploitation be understood in the context of global markets in organs and reproductive services? In answering this question I draw on Snyder's taxonomy of three forms of exploitation (2008, 2012) and Panitch's (2013, 2017) analysis of exploitation in transnational surrogacy contracts.

In a discussion of exploitation in human subject trials of pharmaceuticals, Snyder distinguishes between micro fairness, macro fairness and mere use or needs

[11] For surrogates, who in the Indian context are typically housed in hostels for the duration of pregnancy, the risks are different: loss of affiliation with family and children, loss of control over their lives for the duration of the pregnancy, and the requirement to emotionally distance themselves from the child they are gestating (for more detailed discussion see Pande 2010, Khader 2013).

[12] For a summary of the ethnographic research with Iranian kidney sellers, see Koplin (2014).

exploitation. He argues that these different forms of exploitation can coexist, but each is tied to different vulnerabilities and different forms of wrongdoing (2012, 252). Micro fairness exploitation occurs when asymmetries in the bargaining position of the parties enables the more advantaged party to skew the benefits of the transaction unfairly in their favour. As I mentioned earlier, some advocates of micro fairness accounts do not think that all such transactional unfairness is wrongful, however. In cases of so-called mutually advantageous exploitation, if the party with less bargaining power nevertheless benefits relative to the position she was in before the transaction, and is capable of consenting to it, then this kind of transaction need not be wrongful. This is the view of exploitation assumed by defenders of markets in organs and gestational surrogacy.

Macro fairness accounts of exploitation object that micro fairness accounts fail to attend to long-term and systemic asymmetries in bargaining power arising from background inequalities and injustices. However, these kinds of long-term and systemic asymmetries create vulnerabilities that should be taken into account in assessing the fairness or otherwise of transactions, and the consent of the disadvantaged party. Further, they give rise to duties on the part of the more advantaged to mitigate the effects of injustice and to reform unjust institutions (Snyder 2012, 256).

Macro fairness accounts are likely to be much more sceptical than micro fairness accounts of the claim that mutually advantageous exploitation is permissible. Panitch (2013, 2017), for example, argues that assessments of whether or not so-called mutually advantageous transnational surrogacy contracts are exploitative must attend to background structural injustices that determine the bargaining positions of the parties. She argues that, given these injustices, it is misleading to focus solely on the share of the benefits to the parties to the contract – which is difficult to do in any case, given the incommensurability of the goods or benefits that accrue to the parties in a surrogacy contract. Rather, "underpayment, or unfairness of benefit sharing, must be assessed not just relative to what the other party to the contract gains but relative to what other people performing the same type of work in other parts of the world receive as compensation" (2103, 332). An inter-contractual comparison between an Indian surrogate and her US counterpart with respect to payment as well as other benefits makes it clear that the Indian surrogate's vulnerability is being exploited. Panitch lists benefits such as "freedom to pursue other interests while under contract, health care, travel and dietary expenses, legal representation, a post-birth opt-out clause, and the potential for a rewarding relationship with the adoptive family" (333).

Additionally, the ethnographic research provides evidence that Indian surrogates are not able to negotiate the terms of the contract. In fact, they are explicitly counselled against attempting to negotiate better terms, and warned that they are replaceable by another woman who would be willing to accept the terms (Pande 2010). They are replaceable precisely because there are so many other poor and desperate women; that is, women who are vulnerable, in both situational and pathogenic senses and who experience insecurity across a range of functionings. Panitch argues that this inability to negotiate the terms of the contract is morally equivalent to an inability to refuse; hence their consent is not genuine or authoritative. On grounds of both inter-contractual unfairness of benefit and failure of genuine consent, the claim that these contracts are not wrongful cannot be sustained.

Snyder's third form of exploitation, "mere use exploitation", is a failure of the Kantian duty of beneficence. Elsewhere, in the context of a discussion of sweatshop labour Snyder terms this form of exploitation "needs exploitation": "Needs Exploitation takes place when an exploiter gains advantage from an exploitee while disregarding shortfalls in the basic needs of the exploitee which the exploiter has a duty to meet" (2008, 390). In other words, rather than acting from the duty of beneficence, which requires us to reduce the other's vulnerability, in needs exploitation one takes advantage of the other's vulnerability and disregards her basic needs. Basic needs here refer to the different dimensions of well-being required to lead a minimally decent human life (395). This notion serves as a normative baseline for what is owed to others who stand to us in particular relations of dependence; thus for example, what is owed by parents to their children, employers to employees, researchers to research participants, the state to its citizens.

Like the macro fairness account, the needs exploitation account will be sceptical of the claim that so-called mutually advantageous exploitation is morally permissible. In the case of transnational markets in organs and reproductive services, even if we assume that a specific transaction does not leave a person worse off than they were before and even if it may marginally improve their situation, the transaction is nevertheless exploitative if, due to background structural inequality and injustice, the person's living conditions are such that their basic needs are not met and will not be met subsequent to the transaction. The question of on whom the duty of beneficence falls in such cases is complex, but the relevant parties will include the state, the medical profession, and organ buyers or prospective parents.

## 11.4 Autonomy and Paternalism

The argument so far has made a case that transnational markets in organs and reproductive services exploit persons who are vulnerable and disadvantaged. What then of the argument made by their defenders that such markets increase the option sets of the desperately poor, thereby enhancing their autonomy, and that prohibitions or restrictions on these markets constitute unwarranted paternalism? In this section of the paper, I draw on a relational and multidimensional analysis of autonomy to show why this kind of argument is flawed. I also endorse a suggestion by Malmqvist (2014), that a group soft paternalist approach to commercial markets in organs (and reproductive services) might be justified.

Elsewhere I have argued that a multidimensional and relational analysis of individual or personal autonomy is helpful for clarifying some of the complex questions about autonomy that arise in non-ideal and practical contexts (see e.g. Mackenzie 2014, 2017). Autonomy is both a capacity and a status concept. While my account acknowledges the normative importance of individual autonomy, it aims to clarify the relational dimensions of both the capacity for autonomy and of agents' autonomy status. In doing so, it makes several claims about the requirements for an adequate conception of autonomy: i) it must be responsive to the facts of human vulnerability and dependency, and the need for social relations of care; ii) it must be premised on a conception of individual identity as embodied, and shaped by intersecting social, cultural, political and historical determinants; iii) it must explain the social constitution and scaffolding of autonomy capacities; iv) it must explain how social oppression, inequality and disadvantage can impair individuals' *capacities* to lead autonomous lives – to different degrees and in different ways in different contexts; v) it must explain the ways that our *status* as autonomous agents is vulnerable to the character of our social relationships and the broader social environment; hence how some persons with the *capacity* for autonomy may fail to be recognised and treated by others as having the *status* of autonomous agents. The account thus combines both internalist and externalist conditions for autonomy.

In my view the concept of autonomy encompasses three distinct but causally interconnected dimensions or axes: self-determination, self-governance and self-authorisation (Mackenzie 2014, 2017). Each dimension should be understood as a matter of degree and domain: a person can be self-determining, self-governing and self-authorising to differing degrees, both at a time and over the course of her life.

To be self-determining is to have the authority and power to exercise both *de jure* and *de facto* control over important domains of one's life (cf. Oshana 2006). This authority and power is a function of the freedoms and opportunities available to a person in her social environment and of her social standing or status. The self-determination axis thus draws attention to externalist requirements for autonomy. In my view, it is difficult to lead a self-determining life in contexts characterised by social relations of domination and subordination, where a person's access to relevant freedoms and opportunities is blocked or restricted, and where her status as autonomous agent is constrained by her position within the social hierarchy. I submit it is also difficult to lead a self-determining life in contexts of extreme disadvantage, characterised by insecurity of functioning and a paucity of genuine opportunities for secure functionings.

To be self-governing is to be able to make and enact decisions that express or cohere with one's practical identity, or one's deeply held values and commitments. This involves introspective and emotional skills for self-understanding and self-definition, rational and imaginative skills to envisage and chart a path between a range of alternative courses of action, and self-control to enact and follow through on one's decisions.[13] Hence, the self-governance axis draws attention to internalist requirements for autonomy. However, in my view self-governance is a relationally constituted capacity. The skills required for self-governance are developed and scaffolded (or not) by an agent's social relationships and broader social environment. Self-determination and self-governance, though conceptually distinct, thus interact causally: the authentic *self* of self-governance, and the development and exercise of

[13] For detailed analysis of the emotional and imaginative skills involved in self-governing agency, see Meyers (1989) and Mackenzie (2000, 2002).

the competences required for *governing* the self, are to a significant degree enabled and/or constrained by external social conditions. This is why restricted freedoms, lack of genuine opportunities for functionings, and socially subordinated status can (but need not always) be internalised and manifest in adaptive preference formation, restricted imaginative horizons, and constricted psychological freedom.

To be self-authorising is to regard oneself as having the normative authority to take ownership of, or responsibility for, one's values, decisions and one's life overall. It also involves regarding oneself as an equal participant in reciprocal accountability relations – as able to account for oneself to others and also to hold others to account. Thinking of oneself in this way involves holding appropriate attitudes of self-respect, self-trust and self-esteem.[14] These psychological attitudes are inherently social, because they are developed and sustained through intersubjective social relations and normative structures and practices of social recognition. One of the insidious effects of social subordination, pathogenic vulnerability or disadvantage is that persistent messages of social inferiority and unworthiness, embedded in everyday social interactions or conveyed through demeaning stereotypes and social scripts, can be internalised in feelings of shame and humiliation, of diminished self-respect, self-trust and self-esteem, and of social invisibility.

The ethnographic research indicates that many of the people recruited as organ sellers or gestational surrogates appear to exercise compromised autonomy across these different dimensions. Their severe impoverishment, vulnerability, insecurity with respect to significant functionings, and lack of genuine opportunities for functionings, compromises their capacities to lead self-determining lives. Domination within patriarchal social and familial structures is an additional constraining factor on surrogates' capacities to lead self-determining lives overall, while their enclosure in hostels for the duration of the pregnancy is an enforced restriction on their freedom of movement and affiliation.

These factors, combined with illiteracy, may also compromise these people's capacities to lead self-governing lives. This is not to deny their capacities for agency, nor is it to suggest that they do not know what is of value to them. A central theme to emerge from the ethnographic research is that one of the main motivations for entering into these transactions is people's sense of obligation to provide and care for their families, as well as the hope of leading a more self-determining life. My argument is rather that illiteracy and insecurity of functioning may impair the development and exercise of some of the skills involved in self-governing agency. The regret expressed by many kidney sellers about their decision, documented in some of the ethnographies, seems to support this claim.

Finally with respect to self-authorisation, a theme that emerges from the ethnographic research with both kidney sellers and surrogates is that social inequality and subordination compromises their sense of themselves as self-authorising agents and renders them vulnerable to coercion, deception and corrupt systems of patronage.

[14] For detailed arguments concerning the importance of these self-affective attitudes for autonomy, see Anderson and Honneth (2005), Benson (1994, 2000), Govier (2003), and Mackenzie (2008).

Surrogates, as discussed already, do not feel authorised to negotiate the conditions of the transaction. Kidney sellers report being duped by unscrupulous brokers, ill-treated by medical professionals and socially shamed and excluded following surgery. Some clearly hope that by selling their kidney to a wealthy person they will acquire a patron who will feel an obligation to provide for them.

In light of these considerations, which are informed by the ethnographic research, the claim that markets in organs and reproductive services add an autonomy-enhancing option to desperate people's choices cannot be sustained.[15] To be autonomy-enhancing, in my view, options need to generate fertile functionings (Wolff and de Shalit 2007, 138), functionings that improve people's capacities to lead more autonomous lives overall. This requires concerted efforts on the part of governments and the international community to create genuine opportunities for functionings, thereby beginning to address the structural injustices that create the conditions in which noxious markets can take root.

In response to the objection that this argument is unjustifiably paternalistic, I want to endorse Malmqvist's (2014) appeal to group soft paternalism in defense of a prohibition on kidney sales. Malmqvist argues that a group soft paternalist approach can be justified as autonomy-promoting in situations where: (i) the option to sell a kidney is potentially harmful to sellers; (ii) the autonomy of a significant number of sellers is compromised; and (iii) it is not desirable or practically feasible to make determinations about whether individual sellers do or do not satisfy the conditions for autonomous choice. Thus, the argument is that even if some individual prospective sellers might satisfy the conditions for autonomy, the justification for group soft paternalism is to protect non-autonomous prospective sellers from harms they have not autonomously chosen (118).

## 11.5 Conclusion

My aim in this paper has been to respond to the claim by defenders of transnational markets in organs and reproductive services that these kinds of market transactions constitute autonomy-enhancing and morally permissible forms of mutual exploitation. I have argued that the claim that this form of mutual exploitation is morally permissible cannot be sustained in light of a vulnerability-based approach to exploitation that is informed by an analysis of disadvantage and that is attentive to structural inequality and injustice. Nor can the claim that such markets are autonomy-enhancing be sustained. Although I have not argued in defense of either

[15] See also Gupta, who argues that the language "of choice" in relation to commercial reproductive services in India is "misused and misplaced"; it is a "myth" because women's agency in this context "cannot be isolated from other areas of life that condition women's agency, such as education, own income, vulnerable position within marital household, gender discrimination, and violence" (2012, 46).

prohibition or regulation, the considerations adduced in this paper support the view that a group soft paternalist policy approach to such markets is morally justifiable.

## References


Anderson, Joel, and Axel Honneth. 2005. Autonomy, Vulnerability, Recognition and Justice. In *Autonomy and the Challenges to Liberalism*, ed. John Christman and Joel Anderson, 127–149. Cambridge: Cambridge University Press.

Benson, Paul. 1994. Free Agency and Self-Worth. *Journal of Philosophy* 91: 650–668.

———. 2000. Feeling Crazy: Self-Worth and the Social Character of Responsibility. In *Relational Autonomy: Feminist Perspectives on Autonomy, Agency and the Social Self*, ed. Catriona Mackenzie and Natalie Stoljar, 72–93. New York: Oxford University Press.

Deveaux, Monique, and Vida Panitch, eds. 2017. *Exploitation: From Practice to Theory*. London: Rowman and Littlefield International.

Fabre, Cecile. 2006. *Whose Body Is It Anyway? Justice and the Integrity of the Person*. Oxford: Oxford University Press.

Govier, Trudy. 2003. Self-Trust, Autonomy, and Self-Esteem. *Hypatia* 8: 99–120.

Gupta, Jyotsna Agnihotri. 2012. Reproductive Biocrossings: Indian Egg Donors and Surrogates in the Globalized Fertility Market. *IJFAB* 5 (1): 25–51.

Hurst, Samia A. 2008. Vulnerability in Research and Health Care; Describing the Elephant in the Room? *Bioethics* 22 (4): 191–202.

Khader, Serene. 2013. Intersectionality and the Ethics of Transnational Commercial Surrogacy. *IJFAB* 6 (1): 68–90.

Koplin, Julian. 2014. Assessing the Likely Harms to Kidney Vendors in Regulated Organ Markets. *The American Journal of Bioethics* 14 (10): 7–18.

Mackenzie, Catriona. 2000. Imagining Oneself Otherwise. In *Relational Autonomy: Feminist Perspectives on Autonomy, Agency and the Social Self*, ed. Catriona Mackenzie and Natalie Stoljar, 124–150. New York: Oxford University Press.

———. 2002. Critical Reflection, Self-Knowledge and the Emotions. *Philosophical Explorations: An International Journal for the Philosophy of Mind and Action* 5 (3): 186–206.

———. 2008. Relational Autonomy, Normative Authority and Perfectionism. *Journal of Social Philosophy* 39: 512–533.

———. 2014. Three Dimensions of Autonomy: A Relational Analysis. In *Autonomy, Oppression and Gender*, ed. Andrea Veltman and James Piper, 15–41. New York: Oxford University Press.

———. 2015. Autonomy. In *Routledge Companion to Bioethics*, ed. John Arras, Elizabeth Felton, and Rebecca Kukla, 277–290. New York/London: Routledge.

———. 2017. Feminist Conceptions of Autonomy. In *Routledge Companion to Feminist Philosophy*, ed. Ann Garry, Serene Khader, and Alison Stone, 515–527. New York/London: Routledge.

Mackenzie, Catriona, Wendy Rogers, and Susan Dodds. 2014. What is vulnerability and why does it matter for moral theory? In *Vulnerability: New Essays in Ethics and Feminist Philosophy*, ed. Rogers Mackenzie, 1–29. New York: Oxford University Press.

Malmqvist, Erik. 2014. Are Bans on Kidney Sales Unjustifiably Paternalistic? *Bioethics* 28 (3): 110–118.

Meyers, Diana. 1989. *Self, Society and Personal Choice*. New York: Columbia University Press.

Moazam, Farhat, Riffat Moazam Zaman, and Aamir M. Jafarey. 2009. Conversations with Kidney Vendors in Pakistan: An Ethnographic Study. *Hastings Center Report* 39 (3): 29–44.

Moniruzzaman, Monir. 2012. 'Living Cadavers' in Bangladesh: Bioviolence in the Human Organ Bazaar. *Medical Anthropology Quarterly* 26 (1): 69–91.

Oshana, Marina. 2006. *Personal Autonomy in Society*. Aldershot: Ashgate.

Pande, Amrita. 2010. Commercial Surrogacy in India: Manufacturing a Perfect Mother-Worker. *Signs: Journal of Women in Culture and Society* 35 (4): 969–991.

Panitch, Vida. 2013. Global Surrogacy: Exploitation to Empowerment. *Journal of Global Ethics* 9 (3): 329–343.

———. 2017. Exploitation and Intimate Labor. In *Exploitation: From Practice to Theory*, ed. Monique Deveaux and Vida Panitch, 119–138. London: Rowman and Littlefield International.

Radcliffe-Richards, Janet. 2007. Selling Organs, Gametes and Surrogacy Services. In *The Blackwell Guide to Medical Ethics*, ed. R. Rhodes, L. Francis, and A. Silvers, 254–268. Malden: Wiley-Blackwell.

Rogers, Wendy, Catriona Mackenzie, and Susan Dodds. 2012. Why Bioethics Needs a Concept of Vulnerability. *IJFAB* 5 (2): 11–38.

Scheper-Hughes, Nancy. 2000. The Global Traffic in Human Organs. *Current Anthropology* 41 (2): 191–224.

———. 2008. Illegal Organ Trade: Global Justice and the Traffic in Human Organs. In *Rainer Gruessner and Enrico Beneditti*, ed. Living Donor Organ Transplants, 106–121. New York: McGraw-Hill.

Snyder, Jeremy. 2008. Needs Exploitation. *Ethical Theory and Moral Practice* 11 (4): 389–405.

———. 2012. Exploitations and their Complications: The Necessity of Identifying the Multiple Forms of Exploitation in Pharmaceutical Trials. *Bioethics* 26 (5): 251–258.

Taylor, James Stacey. 2002. Autonomy, constraining options, and organ sales. *Journal of Applied Philosophy* 19 (3): 273–285.

Wertheimer, Alan. 1996. *Exploitation*. Princeton: Princeton University Press.

———. 2011. *Rethinking the Ethics of Clinical Research: Widening the Lens*. New York: Oxford University Press.

Wilkinson, Stephen. 2003. The Exploitation Argument Against Commercial Surrogacy. *Bioethics* 17 (2): 169–187.

Wolff, Jonathon, and Avner de Shalit. 2007. *Disadvantage*. Oxford: Oxford University Press.

# Chapter 12
# Outlook

**James F. Childress and Michael Quante**

Our introduction announced that the chapters in this volume deliver important contributions to ongoing debates about the characterization of personal autonomy and autonomous decisions and actions. Without exaggeration, we can claim that the wide-ranging papers in this book illuminatingly address questions that have been dealt with in many ethical theories for a long time and that elicit concern in numerous social contexts and practices too.

It is also noteworthy that these contributions stem from a specialized philosophical context, namely, analytic philosophy, and that they mostly focus on problems and questions related to biomedical ethics or bioethics (in a fairly broad sense) and ethics more generally. In the last few decades, in modern western societies, respect for autonomy has become the most important, or at least one of the most dominant, ethical principles. In addressing (and countering) paternalism in many dis-guises, our practices and social contexts have changed in many ways. Another effect is that many ethical theories rely on thin conceptions of personal autonomy and some even limit their focus to decisions or actions. Many authors presuppose that only minimal, formal, or procedural conceptions of autonomy can adequately protect individuals from paternalism.

In the last three decades, concerns have emerged about the limitations of such thin conceptions. The dialectic of this debate has led to the reemergence of "thick" conceptions of various kinds. These make explicit the anthropological, biographical, and social aspects of our being human persons. Because autonomy and living one's life as a person are interrelated in various ways, these have enriched our

J. F. Childress
University of Virginia, Charlottesville, VA, USA
e-mail: jfc7c@virginia.edu

M. Quante (✉)
University of Münster, Münster, Germany
e-mail: michael.quante@uni-muenster.de



J. F. Childress, M. Quante (eds.), *Thick (Concepts of) Autonomy*, Philosophical Studies Series 146, https://doi.org/10.1007/978-3-030-80991-1_12

conceptions of autonomy. As the chapters in our volume demonstrate, this has implications for the ethical requirement to respect autonomy as an ethical principle on the one hand and within many social practices on the other.

Against this background, this volume offers a wide range of perspectives. Its chapters explicate the central elements of and the many relations between "thin" and "thick" concepts of autonomy and identify normative and social consequences these different conceptions might (or actually do) have in our practices. These chapters demonstrate the importance of these matters for ethics and biomedical ethics.

Nevertheless, it remains true that the contributions in our volume are located within a specialized discourse in analytic practical philosophy and biomedical ethics. No single volume can address all the contexts in which autonomy is rooted and important or analyze all dimensions of autonomy—needless to say, such a task would also be far beyond our competences. Here, we only briefly outline three contexts to open wider perspectives and to identify areas for further research and scholarly debate.

## 12.1 Other Philosophical Traditions

"Autonomy" is a term of art; therefore, we cannot use ordinary language or our daily uses of the term as a source and corrective for our analysis. Moreover, the term is rooted in different scholarly and scientific disciplines. This means that the concepts and conceptions of autonomy are differently framed in different disciplines (sometimes even in different schools or traditions within a single discipline). Because "autonomy" is not a natural kind we have to accept that different concepts or conceptions are meaningful in light of different epistemic interests or premises (e.g. concerning methods).

Furthermore, the concept of autonomy has a long and complex history sedimented in etymology. In ancient Greece, it was used mainly in the context of political philosophy, where it referred to the right of a political entity (e.g. a polis) to rule its inner affairs without external influence. In modern times, and especially in the philosophy of Rousseau and Kant, the concept of autonomy was transferred from political entities to human agents. Since then, it has stood for a human's capacity for self-determination and for the perfectionist ideal to realize this capacity both in one's individual life and in one's social context. In the romantic tradition, autonomy also became important in philosophical aesthetics, where it was enriched by such concepts as originality, authenticity, and expressing one's (real) self. Altogether, autonomy became embedded in at least three philosophical language games:

- autonomy and responsibility (two main foci on human agency in ethics)
- autonomy and freedom (a main metaphysical theme in action theory)
- autonomy and personhood (a central relation in both theoretical and practical philosophy)

The volume of literature in analytic philosophy and in the broader western tradition is unmanageable in each of these three contexts. In each one, autonomy is juxtaposed to specific conceptual 'counterparts' (e.g. autonomy vs. authenticity in the third or autonomy vs. autarky in the second). In addition, the concept of autonomy is analyzed against the background of specific types of philosophy; for example, in ethics, the explication is different within a deontological framework than within a utilitarian meta-ethics. The chapters in this volume provide evidence for this multi-layered and complex structure of the concept of autonomy in the western tradition of philosophy and within the narrower tradition of analytic philosophy.

Therefore, in a wider perspective, the concept of autonomy should be analyzed in relation to alternative traditions in analytic philosophy (e.g. the late Wittgenstein and his followers) or in western philosophy (e.g. German idealism or pragmatism). Some of the themes and topics developed there have left their traces in contributions to this volume that try to overcome weaknesses of thin conceptions of autonomy (e.g. Christman or Mackenzie) by bringing into view the social dimension of agency and personhood.

In an even wider perspective of intercultural philosophy, the western tradition (of which this book only covers a small part) needs to be compared and contrasted with other conceptions of agency and the self (e.g. in Asian or African traditions). This would be relevant not only for a comprehensive analysis of concepts of autonomy in all philosophical traditions. It will also be practically important in all pluralistic social contexts in which respect for autonomy functions as a normative resource. For example, the more biomedical ethics deals with diverse and multicultural settings, the more urgently it will need to understand sociocultural differences in interpretations of autonomy.

## 12.2 Changing Environments

Our societies are characterized by dynamic changes in technologies and social structures. In both contexts, the concept of autonomy and the principle of respect for autonomy need to be rethought and further developed. In an aging society, living wills become an important tool to extend one's autonomy along with diverse artificial assistance systems in long-term care or in the care of persons with dementia. Information technologies, big data, and new forms of mass communication (e.g. via twitter et al.) all raise questions about how to spell out autonomy in data ethics or informational self-control. And these changes will have consequences for all of us as politically responsible agents too.

Even more complicated issues lurk in the field of artificial systems that are regarded as autonomous agents themselves. Our everyday conceptions of autonomy and responsibility are prominently challenged by autonomous driving and, less prominently but significantly, by smart weapons. We have to ask: Do such tools preserve or strengthen our autonomous actions? Or do they replace our autonomy by taking away our responsibility?

Finally, some developments seem to destroy autonomy from the outset by using enhancement technologies as tools for self-optimizing our bodily and psychological capacities. Perhaps moral enhancement is a good idea from the viewpoint of an educator interested in the good. But can such a replacement of normal human autonomy still be regarded as a version of our autonomy? From the perspectives in this volume, it is evident that the concept of autonomy itself has too many dimensions and appears in too many contexts and traditions to function as a safe anchor. Evaluating these dynamics requires a much broader set of philosophical tools as we seek to determine whether these developments are strengthening, transforming, or destroying our autonomy.

## 12.3 Intra- and Interdisciplinary Contexts

Facing this complexity is both philosophically fascinating and threatening. Obviously it cannot be addressed adequately within one single book or by one philosopher alone. Like agency, personhood, and free will, the conception of autonomy is a topic for different sub-disciplines in philosophy (intra-disciplinarity) and needs to be dealt with through interdisciplinary cooperation.

Within philosophy itself, with its widely accepted subdisciplines, it is evident that philosophy of action and person, epistemology, and ethics need to be integrated (even in thin conceptions). In any adequate analysis of thick conceptions, philosophical anthropology and political and social philosophy also will become central. Some of this intradisciplinary dialectic operates in the contributions of our volume. Others would become visible if we were to widen the philosophical perspective beyond the tradition of analytic philosophy featured in this book.

Finally, empirical research (e.g., in psychology or sociology) is important for understanding and using the concept of autonomy in real life and social practices. Our understanding and use also need to be enriched by scientific knowledge and evidence from cultural anthropology, biology, and medicine. In some contexts (e.g. illness, human embodiment, aging, or dying), medical knowledge is central, but much more is needed. This is especially the case when we recognize the cultural framing of these anthropologically basic features of our human existence.

Autonomy is a central and distinctive feature of our *lebensform*. Since human persons are complex and dynamic entities, they must be considered from a variety of perspectives — within and beyond philosophy. In this volume, we offer one way into this complex phenomenon; we also aim at making accessible some of the complexities and tensions surrounding autonomy. But we do not pretend to deliver an exhaustive or even a comprehensive analysis of personal autonomy. This we couldn't have willed autonomously—it would be far beyond what we can do. The limits of the philosophical debates represented in this volume should be taken as motivation, as a challenging opportunity for further multidisciplinary and interdisciplinary discussion to enrich our understanding of what it means to be autonomous human persons in the world.

# Index





J. F. Childress, M. Quante (eds.), *Thick (Concepts of) Autonomy*, Philosophical Studies Series 146, https://doi.org/10.1007/978-3-030-80991-1

The manufacturer's authorised representative in the EU is Springer Nature Customer Service Centre GmbH, Europaplatz 3, 69115 Heidelberg, Germany. If you have any concerns regarding our products, please contact ProductSafety@springernature.com

Printed and bound by CPI Group (UK) Ltd, Croydon, CR0 4YY
30/09/2026
02225690-0003